THE ATHLETE AFTER

A 10-Week Guide to Balancing Life After Sports

Katie Hargrave
Holistic Health Coach & Personal Trainer

Copyright © 2016 by Katie Hargrave

All rights reserved. No part of this book may be reproduced in any form or by any electronic or mechanical means, including information storage and retrieval systems, without permission in writing from the author. For information, contact Katie Hargrave by visiting athleteafterword.com.

The content of this book is for general informational purposes only. It is not meant to be used, nor should it be used, to diagnose or treat any medical condition or to replace the services of your physician or other health care provider. The advice and strategies contained in the book may not be suitable for all readers. Please consult your health care provider for any questions that you may have about your own medical situation. Neither the author, publisher, IIN® nor any of their employees or representatives guarantees the accuracy of information in this book or its usefulness to a particular reader, nor are they responsible for any damages or negative consequences that may result from any treatment, action taken, or inaction by any person reading or following the information in this book.

Back cover photo: Nellie Shots Photography

ISBN-10: 1539873129
ISBN-13: 978-1539873129

ABOUT THE AUTHOR

Katie Hargrave has her Holistic Health Coaching certification from the Institute for Integrative Nutrition®, and is a member of the International Association for Health Coaches (IAHC). She is also a Certified Personal Trainer through the American Council on Exercise (ACE). She was a competitive athlete for 15 years, finishing her basketball career in 2011the NCAA Division II level at Saint Martin's University in Lacey, Washington. She realized at that time she didn't know how to eat or exercise when it wasn't for her sport. She spent several years researching and trying different programs until she was able to find what worked for her. Through the process, she realized her passion is helping others in their journey of finding balanced health.

Katie is currently living in Olympia, Washington. Rather than offering a set nutritional and/or training program for everyone, Katie takes the time to understand each individual's needs, help in goal development, as well as providing strategies and support to achieve success. Whether for health coaching, personal training, or both, Katie provides assistance with weight loss, maintenance, or muscle gain; increased energy and quality of sleep; as well as help in understanding your relationship with food and exercise, and which foods and activities are right for you.

In addition to working with individuals, Katie is also a speaker to parents and teams about nutritional guidelines for athletes. To learn more about Katie and her work, visit her website at athleteafterword.com or Facebook Page at facebook.com/athleteafter.

This book was chosen as a winner of the Launch Your Dream Book Top 10 Author Contest through the Institute for Integrative Nutrition.

"The Athlete After is written by Katie Hargrave, a graduate of the Institute for Integrative Nutrition, where they completed a cutting edge curriculum in nutrition and health coaching taught by the world's leading experts in health and wellness. I recommend you read this book and be in touch with Katie Hargrave to see how she can help you successfully achieve your goals."

- Joshua Rosenthal, MScEd,
Founder/Director, Institute for Integrative Nutrition

ACKNOWLEDGMENTS

I would like to thank everyone who supported me in putting this book together, and who helped it come into fruition. Thank you to my husband, Matt Hargrave, for supporting me in taking the course that led to this book's publication. I also would like to acknowledge those who took the time to read through my manuscript and provide helpful feedback: Matt Hargrave, Jamey Schoeneberg, Beth Olson, Karli Kirk, Misty Suggs, David Millen, and Dr. Tom Helpenstell. Thank you Nellie Heay for helping me find my good angles in our search for a good headshot; as well as Shannon McMillan for helping me create a beautiful cover.

TABLE OF CONTENTS

Introduction 1
    How to Read This Book 8

Food 17
    You Are What You Eat 19
    Water 20
    Macronutrients 21
    Protein 22
    Carbohydrates 30
    Fat 35
    How Our Bodies Use Food for Energy 41
    Overall Calorie Intake 43
    Micronutrients and Nutrient Density 43
    Nutrition and the Mind 48
    Putting it all Together 49

Body 51
    Post-Sport Exercise 53
    Excess Exercise: Stress and the Body 53
    How Much Exercise is Enough? 56
    What Type of Athlete Are You? 58
    Exercising with Chronic Issues 62
    Accepting Your Body 64
    Mind-Body Connection 66

Mind 71
    Identity: I Am an Athlete 73
    Changing Focus 74
    Getting What You Want: Meditation & Setting Intentions 77
    The Change in Relationships 81
    Additional Support 82

Univera: Essential Products 87
Becoming a Health Coach 89
References 91
Transition Plan 97

INTRODUCTION

For as long as you can remember, your focus has been on the next win. Push harder. Go faster. Get stronger. You endure long practices. You juggle tryouts, tournaments, and travel. You skip holidays, gatherings, and parties to train, compete, and succeed. You live with the pressure to get the next win, earn a scholarship, and be the best. More reps, more shots, more drills—you do anything to gain the edge. "Somewhere out there, someone is training harder," every coach says.

Then all of a sudden, whether planned or not, it's done. Years of work, years of sacrifice, and years of competing—literally, years of blood, sweat, and tears—come to a conclusion. They say an athlete dies twice, the first being when they retire.

There is no doubt that the termination of a career in sports is a significant time in an athlete's life. The adjustment includes a change not only in nutrition and exercise, but also in self-perception, social environment, emotions, and relationships.

Given the significance of athletic retirement, researchers have begun to examine it as a life event rather than a single event.[1] Scholars now believe that to understand athletic retirement in its entirety, it is imperative to view the process from the time one starts playing to post-sport participation.[2]

The four most common reasons why athletes part ways with

---

[1] Blinde and Greendorfer, "A reconceptualization of the process of leaving the role of competitive athlete"; Wylleman, Alfermann and Lavallee, "Career transitions in sport."
[2] Oglivie and Lavallee, "Career transition among athletes."

their sport are age, de-selection, injury, and free choice.² It has been shown that athletes who end their careers expectedly (foreseen retirement due to graduation or on their own terms) are much more likely to have an easier transition than those who suffer a career-ending injury or who fail to make a team. However, even those who know the end-date of their athletic career may go through the five stages of grief: denial, anger, bargaining (if only I had…), depression, and acceptance.

Athletes who suffer a career-ending injury are more likely to experience grief, identity loss, loneliness, anxiety and fear, loss of confidence, depression, alcohol abuse, and even suicide.³ They report lower life satisfaction five to ten years following retirement compared to those who were not injured.⁴ However, while injury-related retirements relinquish a sense of control, the athlete is spared the message that they weren't good enough, which could otherwise lead to decreased self-esteem and self-confidence.⁵

College athletes who believed they would obtain a professional sports career, but who did not, also had lower life satisfaction and self-esteem after college compared to those who planned on moving into a different field after graduation.⁵ When evaluating their experience after college, those who believed they would play professionally showed lower self-perceived success in school, less participation in class, a lower grade point average,

---

[3] D. Alfermann et all, "Causes and consequences of sport career termination"; P. Lally, "Identity and athletic retirement"; Pearson and Petitpas, "Transitions of athletes."

[4] Kleiber and Brock, "The effect of career-ending injuries on the subsequent well-being of elite college athletes."

[5] Smith and McManus, "A Review on Transitional Implications for Retiring Elite Athletes."

and less perceived value of education because they were more invested in their sport.[4]

In reality, the chances of becoming a professional athlete are extremely low. A 2016 study underscores this statement, noting that the odds of playing professional football is one in 4,233; men's soccer one in 5,768; men's basketball one in 11,771; and women's basketball one in 13,015.[6] In addition to these discouraging odds, professional sport opportunities are extremely short term. The average career in a team sport lasts between three to seven years,[7] leaving approximately 40 additional years in a person's work life.

Professional athletes are also portrayed as wealthy individuals with an unlimited income. However, salaries vary widely, and super contract athletes are the rare exception. Most participants sign for the league minimum and are often forced out of their career for various reasons before they can cash out.[7] For example, in 2014, a group of minor league baseball players sued the MLB because the league didn't even pay them minimum wage, with salaries as low as $5,500 per year.[7] The MLB justifies it by classifying it as seasonal pay, and minor league players are not paid for any offseason training they do to keep in shape.[7] As for the NFL, beyond any guaranteed bonuses, their contracts are largely not guaranteed. Unlike some other sports, if an NFL player gets cut before completing the contracted amount of time, they can also lose their salary.[7]

Those who do make large amounts of money do not

---

[6] "The Odds of Success."

[7] Marissa Payne, "So you want to be a pro athlete?"

necessarily plan ahead. They often overlook the taxes they must pay in each state they play, neglect saving money to pay for healthcare to repair their bodies once they retire, fail to recognize they must continue to make payments on large mortgages, and bypass the need to spread their earnings over the rest of their lifetime.

The Transition

Chances are if you are reading this, you are in some way dealing with the aftermath of your retirement, or you are preparing for it. Even if you think you are ready, it is a huge change, and a close to a significant chapter in your life.

That's how the transition was for me. Between the ages of seven and nine, my parents started me in several sports—softball, soccer, and basketball. With some height, and a bit of athletic ability, basketball was my strong suit. Before long, it had become the primary focus of my young athletic life. By the time I entered seventh grade, I was playing year-round elite basketball with a tournament almost every weekend, plus school athletics. There was never a season when I wasn't playing at least one sport.

My parents pushed me—hard. The overall goal was to get a scholarship. Until the moment I signed my letter committing to my university of choice, it seemed every decision I made, or that was made for me, hinged on propelling me towards this goal.

When I signed with Saint Martin's University in Lacey, Washington, a private Division II school, it felt like the right fit. I liked the university's small class sizes, which suggested I would get a quality education to use in my future career choice (I had woken up to the fact that I wasn't going to make it to the WNBA). I did not have to take summer school classes to make up for the low number of credits taken during my sporting season, as is often the case with many Division I athletes. However, the rest of my time at Saint Martin's University resembled a typical collegiate sport experience. I often missed class, endured two-hour practices followed by weight lifting, played a tournament on Thanksgiving, had two to three days off for Christmas, and had to balance a full time class load with my sport. Many of us also had the daunting task of juggling jobs, clubs, and extra-curricular activities.

Experiences such as these teach an athlete how to work well as part of a team, strive hard for success, and develop effective time management skills, along with uncountable valuable lessons. However, they do not teach the athlete how to be healthy once their sport experience concludes (or even how to be healthy while in the midst of it all).

In my experience, I did not anticipate having any problem with the transition. In fact, I was all too ready to say goodbye to the activity that had consumed my life for so long. After my last game, I threw away my shoes, practice jerseys, and pretty much anything that remained in my locker. I was ready for something different.

However, I still had difficulty transitioning into the "real world," especially when it came to nutrition and exercise. I decided I was in need of well-deserved break from exercising and went on a six-month hiatus. Yet, I made no change to my eating habits. I continued to live on a diet of frozen pizzas, boxed food that I could easily make myself, and fast food. I had never learned how to cook. My mom had given me a pass because I was always consumed with sports.

I, of course, gained weight quickly. After 20 pounds, I looked in the mirror and couldn't believe I was struggling to keep weight off. I never had to worry about this before. In response, I threw myself back in the gym for two hours per day and starved myself to get my weight back down. Then, when I reached my goal, I was so exhausted and hungry I went right back to sitting on the couch with a pint of ice cream. The yo-yo dieting cycle continued. At about the point when I started having thoughts about using laxatives and even throwing up to lose the weight, I realized I had a problem—and I wasn't the only one.

I started to notice that, like me, many of my fellow former college athletes were having trouble adjusting to a reality that didn't include their sport full time. I observed other burned out athletes who quit exercising completely and gained an unhealthy amount of weight; beautiful women who reacted to the change in their bodies by developing eating disorders to achieve their "competition" size; and several who suffered a career-ending injury slip into depression.

On top of nutrition and exercise issues, I was having trouble in my career of choice. I originally sought a career in publishing, but quickly found that sitting at a desk in front of a computer all day was not for me. I needed a team—a team to work with and influence others, to set goals with, and to see results. I needed to be around like-minded people who I could identify with, and who desired activity and a healthy lifestyle. I needed to achieve success and be recognized.

I struggled with my career choice, identity, nutrition, and exercise after concluding a sport that was, for more than 15 years, my primary life focus. How do you adjust to a new lifestyle when being a basketball player, football player, swimmer, runner, etc., is no longer your identity? How do you eat? How do you exercise when you don't have to be in peak physical condition at all times? How do you become comfortable in a changing body? After following my own path to balanced health and finding myself, I realized I wanted to help other athletes through this transition.

Interestingly, people often don't think athletes should have a problem transitioning and, even in the midst of it all, many currently competing athletes don't think there will be difficulty maintaining health after retirement. Athletes by nature are mentally tough individuals; and, they are often perceived by the rest of society to be fitter, healthier, and happier than others. Due to this belief, there aren't many resources to help a post-sport athlete.

Aside from exploring what influences a positive or negative transition out of sports, limited research has been done on the broader psychological, social, and physical adjustments athletes experience after concluding their career.[5] While some institutions offer support services in preparation for the post-sport life transition, the majority are geared towards an athlete's immediate performance and academic goals. Many lack depth in areas such as general social skills, self-esteem and resiliency skills, and coping strategies for lifestyle changes.[5] In the case of professional sports, the institution's support often ceases immediately upon retirement. Support for college athletes may conclude upon graduation.[5] In either case, once an institution's support has ended, athletes are left to navigate an unfamiliar lifestyle on their own.

The earlier you can begin preparing for this transition by planning for alternative career paths, building social circles outside of athletics, and developing an understanding of nutrition and exercise, the easier retirement will be. My goal for this book is to provide a tool to support athletes preparing for or struggling with the transition out of their sport.

How to Read This Book

This book is broken out into three general sections to help the post-sport athlete navigate the transition to balanced health: food, body, and mind.

The sections are set up in the way that was most helpful to me during my own transition, as well as what has worked best for my clients. Listening to your body is one of the most important ways of understanding your own health, and therefore a natural starting point. Once you start eating clean, you will become much more aware of how different types of foods affect you physically and mentally.

Next, it is important to gain an understanding of how exercise differs when one is training for competition versus working to attain a healthy and balanced lifestyle. In my experience, many athletes feel they should have a good handle on how to exercise since they have been doing it the majority of their life. However, goals change—and how to exercise and find motivation to reach those goals differ. Perhaps you were a soccer player who now wants to try your hand at triathlons.

THE ATHLETE AFTER

How do you train for these new goals? What will your motivation be now that you don't have to meet a coach's expectation? Or, perhaps now you want to understand how to work out to maintain a healthy lifestyle rather than training for anything specific. How do you find balance?

After gaining an understanding of what food and activity the body needs, the next step is to dig deeper into the shift of identity. Many athletes identify themselves primarily as such, and upon retirement are left asking the question, "who am I, now?" Others who realize our lives have changed may nonetheless expect the same levels of performance and achievement we enjoyed as athletes. For those who spent most of their life with a primary focus on their sport, it can be difficult to live up to these expectations.

Although this progression has worked for many of my clients, it doesn't necessarily mean this is what will work for each person. I encourage athletes to focus on what they are struggling with most as a starting point, and move on from there.

For the transitioning athlete, this information may seem overwhelming at first. After all, this transition is possibly the biggest change in an athlete's life. Focusing on one step at a time can help make this change less daunting, and will give you more time to develop lifelong and sustainable habits. To guide this process, included at the end of the book is a space for you to consider the advice given in each section and form your own, personalized 10-week transition plan. I highly suggest giving yourself a full week for each step. I generally work with clients on three- to six-month programs to ensure they have enough time to feel and implement change, so 10 weeks is already moving very quickly! To gain a better idea of what's ahead, I've summarized each section.

Food

One would assume that athletes who play sports at an elite level would receive coaching on nutrition, such as what a growing athlete should eat, or what an athlete should eat before and after practice or competition. I never received this help, and my parents didn't know either.

As a young athlete, I had no real control over what food was available to me. I was sick often, and would vomit at least once per week after practice. At the time, I thought this was normal—after all, I was working hard in conditioning. My coaches criticized me for being too skinny, and told me to bulk up. Yet, when my parents asked them what I should be eating, they had no concrete suggestions.

When I got to college, I was given more direction on proper weight lifting techniques. However, I was still not given direction on what and how to eat. My teammates and I were left to eat whatever we wanted. Luckily, with a cafeteria, there were many more options available. The only time any information was provided was when it became obvious that several of my teammates weren't eating enough. Only then were we handed a packet of information and given a 15-minute talk on how many calories we should be consuming. I barely even knew how to read a food label. Plus, I could barely afford to eat anything other than boxed pasta. Later it became apparent that many colleges, especially outside of Division I athletic programs, weren't supporting or educating athletes on what they should be eating—let alone how they should adjust when they are finished.

Typically, once an athlete is no longer playing their sport, they continue eating the same foods. It's often all they've ever known, and many athletes are used to being able to maintain a good physique while still eating whatever they want. As a result, this is usually how they continue to eat when they retire.

Additionally, many athletes don't think much about food while in their sport because they know it doesn't change the way they look. Student-athletes may be so busy that they rarely think about food at all, and therefore barely eat enough to sustain them through class—let alone practice or competition. Then when they do remember to eat, it's typically something fast and unhealthy. What they fail to realize is how much it can change their athletic performance, strength, and focus.

Without a shift in food choices and amount, there is typically unwanted weight gain. Not only is the change in their physique a shock to the athlete, but suddenly many have joined the rest of the population, which is at risk for chronic disease and part of the very real obesity epidemic. According to the Centers for Disease Control and Prevention, as of 2016:

- 69 percent of American adults (age 20 and older) are over weight or obese. **That's more than two in three adults.**
- This is the first generation of children that is not expected to outlive their parents.
- Chronic diseases and conditions related to obesity—such as heart disease, stroke, cancer, diabetes, and arthritis—are among the most common, costly, and preventable of all health problems.

- The estimated annual medical cost of obesity in the U.S. is between $147-210 billion per year; the medical costs for people who are obese were $1,429 higher than those of normal weight.

All of a sudden we face the fact that we are fighting these statistics like everyone else.

So, what do you do? This section covers the general differences between what athletes should eat to support their activity, and what retired athletes should do to maintain an appropriate weight and balanced health when they are no longer spending hours in the gym every day. In your Transition Plan, you will be experimenting with this information and taking note of how you feel to find which food combinations work best for your body. This is called "bio-individuality™." What may work for me may not be the best foods for you. This is a key area of emphasis—it is crucial to figure out what makes each individual thrive.

Body

When it comes to exercise, it's typical for athletes to do one of two things when they retire: go on a gym strike because "they deserve a break" (that was me); or, continue to exercise two to three hours per day because "it isn't worth going to the gym for any less time" (that was me after I gained weight from doing the first thing).

Many of you, like me, may have done both: took a break, gained weight, and went back to the gym, not knowing how to exercise to reach new goals. Strangely enough, not knowing how to work out in any way other than my sport was a challenge. As a post player I had been trained to lift for bulk; however, after I finished I wanted a leaner physique. The trouble was I didn't know how to lift any other way. All of a sudden I wasn't following a provided plan. I didn't know what exercises to do or why. Nor did I know how many repetitions to do. I often wandered around the gym doing random lifts, then I would get on the treadmill or elliptical for 45 minutes. My local gym offered a free consultation with a trainer, but I felt like I shouldn't need a trainer because I'd been working out for years and, as a collegiate athlete, I should know what to do. Sound familiar?

Looking back, I wish I had started working with a trainer in college, or earlier. Not only would off-season guidance have helped me to lift correctly and better equip me to reach my goals in my specific position, but the feedback on muscular imbalances would have also helped prevent injuries. Only when I started my own personal training certification program did I really start understanding my body and how to reach my specific goals. Consulting with a trainer can help refocus post-sport athletes on new goals and give them the tools to achieve their desired outcome, whether it is building endurance versus strength, or losing weight versus building muscle, etc.

Developing a balanced exercise routine also comes from knowing how your body responds after different types of workouts. How much time per week do you spend on cardio? Yoga? Circuit training? This section will help you figure out what works best for your schedule and your post-sport body, as well as help you to accept your body and appreciate it for what it is and what it's done for you. In your Transition Plan you will be making exercise goals and track how your body feels as you do different types of activity—again, honing in on what works best for your body. You will also be taken through some exercises to help with self love and positivity.

Mind

Successful athletes are mentally strong. They have to be to hit game-winning free throws, take constructive criticism from a coach screaming in their faces, and believe in their team when no one else does. Athletes have been coached on how to visualize, prepare for competition, and block out all distractions. So, why aren't we applying these same strategies to the rest of our lives?

Being mentally strong also doesn't equate to an easier mental transition. In fact, the more we identify as an athlete, the more difficult the transition is.

Most of us think we are prepared for the change in career, especially if we are transitioning out of collegiate sports. However, I'll warn you that in your new place of work, all of a sudden you will not be the "athlete" any more. Chances are no one knows about your athletic skills and achievements, and no one is going to be giving you any special treatment. You have to earn respect, albeit in a different way than you've had to before. The way people identify you changes, and, eventually, the way you identify yourself.

In an effort to help the athlete transition into a new career, various organizations have recently made strides in athlete support. The International Olympic Committee launched its Athlete Career Programme in 2005, Team USA started its Athlete Career and Education Program in 2014, the National Football League now offers a Career Transition Program, and the National Collegiate Athletic Association (NCAA) has an After the Game Career Center. However, these resources, and many others, often just help with employment and fail to recognize the need for emotional support, as well as nutritional and physical adaptation.

Most programs also seem to largely target elite athletes who are still competing. Little attention is directed to recently retired athletes who find themselves at an "in-between" place. This is a crucial time for continued intervention to influence the quality and development of an athlete into post-sport life, and prevent difficulties associated with the transition.[8]

Even if you don't have adequate resources or support during your transition, you don't have to feel lost. You can channel the strengths you've gained from athletics into your new career, and identify with those strengths, instead of identifying yourself as "an athlete." This section will help you understand these strengths and how to utilize them to reach new goals. Ultimately, it will help you figure out what career is best for you as an individual. (Hint: it may not be what you thought—and that's OK!)

---

[8] Stephan, et al., "Repercussions of transition out of elite sport on subjective well-being: a one year study."

FOOD

You Are What You Eat

Chances are, unless you competed professionally or at the Division I level, you didn't get much guidance on what you were supposed to eat as an elite athlete. Crazy, right? I mean, don't you think it's important we understand that which literally fuels us and gives us energy to perform?

> **TRANSITION PLAN**
> *Week One - Food Tracking*
> Start noting your food intake this week. This will allow you to observe your starting point.

Even if you were fortunate enough to receive nutritional support about what and how to eat while competing, chances are even more likely you never received help with what and how to eat when you are done. If you haven't figured it out by now, it's different. Especially if you were an "I'll just burn it off" person. Eating whatever you want won't fly when you work 9-5 p.m. at a desk and then come home to make your own food, and possibly take care of others.

In either scenario, some competitive athletes may not be interested in learning about nutrition since they are still able to stay lean and fit no matter what they take in. This is a huge mistake. Just because you can eat it and not gain weight, doesn't mean that it is good for you, fueling you properly, and helping you to perform the best you can. The "I'll just burn it off" mentality is a set-up for failure—not only does everything you put in your mouth affect you at a cellular level, but it's also allowing you to develop horrible habits that stick with you once you stop working out constantly. Luckily, more parents, coaches, and athletes are understanding the importance of food and seeking out support and information.

So, how do nutritional requirements change? Let's start with what the general athlete should be drinking and eating. Of course, there will be differences depending on what type of athlete you are: a long distance runner is going to eat differently than a sprinter, and a football player eats differently than a gymnast. Everyone is an individual and has specific needs that need to be met in order for them feel their best.

Water

Did you know that your body is made up of between 60 to 75 percent water? It's no surprise how important water is to our health. Too much water can result in mineral imbalances, while too little water can cause dehydration, headaches, and fatigue.

> **TRANSITION PLAN**
> *Week Two - Water*
> Focus on tracking your water intake and trying to get the amount that is right for you.

Water flushes toxins out of vital organs and carries nutrients to your cells. The Institute of Medicine determined that an adequate intake (AI) for men is roughly about 13 cups (3 liters) of total beverages a day. The AI for women is about 9 cups (2.2 liters) of total beverages a day.[9] You may have also heard the general rule of eight, eight-ounce glasses per day (64 ounces total). It's not too far off, and easy to remember—it is typically what I recommend as a goal for those who struggle with water intake.

---

[9] "Water: How Much Should You Drink Every Day?"

However, it is important to note the amount of water a person needs differs by individual, and is affected by factors such as size, activity level, climate, health status, or pregnancy. If you are sweating (active or due to environmental factors), sick, or pregnant/breast feeding, you need more water to make up for what is lost. While there are specific guidelines for each of these scenarios, another easy way to remember what to aim for above the eight glasses a day is to drink half your body weight in ounces. That means someone who weighs 165 pounds would target drinking between 64 to 83 ounces of water per day.

An easy way to measure how much you drink is to carry around a water bottle and take note of how many ounces it holds. If you are shooting for about 80 ounces of water per day, you would then know you need to refill your 20 oz. water bottle four times to reach your goal.

If you start to notice you are getting headaches and craving salt, you may be drinking too much water and flushing out your electrolytes. Start taking note of how you feel, and adjust.

Macronutrients

Food supplies the body with both nutrients and calories. All calories come from macronutrients: proteins, carbohydrates, and fats.

Protein

Protein is the building block of all tissues in the body, including muscle. A protein is made up of amino acids, which help our bodies grow, repair body tissue, and perform many bodily functions. There are 20 different amino acids. Your body is capable of synthesizing half of these on its own (Unessential Amino Acids). The other half must be consumed through dietary sources (Essential Amino Acids).

Most typically know they get protein from animal sources, such as egg whites, steak, and chicken. But, did you know there are many vegetarian and vegan sources as well?

Examples of Animal Protein

Meat	Chicken, turkey, duck, lamb, beef, buffalo, and game.
Eggs	Quick, practical, and inexpensive. The egg white is where the protein can be found, and the yokes carry healthy fats.
Dairy	Milk, cheese, yogurt, and butter. Buy organic to avoid bovine growth hormone and antibiotics.
Fish	A lean, healthy source. Oily fish (salmon, tuna, sardines, etc.) contain heart and brain-healthy omega-3s. Eat fish lower on the food chain (like sardines) to help decrease the risk of mercury and other toxins, and avoid fish that is genetically engineered and/or farmed.
Seafood	Crab, shrimp, oysters, prawns, and lobster.

Examples of Plant Protein

Grains	Brown rice, quinoa, buckwheat, and oats.
Beans	Black, pinto, garbanzo, chickpeas, lentil, mung, and kidney. Beans contain a more complete set of amino acids than other plant foods.
Soy	Common forms of soy beans include edamame, tofu, tempeh, and miso. Today, soy comes in various, unnatural and highly processed forms, like commercial soy milk, soy meat, and soy ice cream. Soy beans are one of the most genetically engineered crops, so try choosing organic when possible.
Nuts	Generally considered a heart-healthy fat, nuts contain protein, fatty acids, fiber, vitamin E, and antioxidants. Peanuts are far higher in protein than other nuts.
Leafy Greens	Broccoli, spinach, kale, collard greens, bok choy, romaine lettuce, and watercress all contain varying amounts of protein. Leafy greens also contain magnesium, iron, and calcium; as well as quercetin, which includes antioxidants, is an anti-inflammatory, and has cancer fighting properties.
Seeds	High in nutrients and lower in caloric content than nuts, seeds provide anti-inflammatory and cardiovascular benefits. Containing vitamin E, fiber, and Omega-3s, some of the healthiest seeds include chia, flax, hemp, pumpkin, sesame and sunflower.

You do not need to eat essential and nonessential amino acids at every meal, but getting a balance of them over the whole day is important. Animal-based foods, such as meat, fish, poultry, dairy products, and eggs, are considered complete proteins because they contain all the essential amino acids. Plant-based foods contain a variety of amino acids, but with the exception of soybeans and quinoa, do not contain all 10 amino acids at once. Such foods are considered incomplete proteins. However, you can form complete proteins by combining different foods together. For instance, you can pair beans with whole grains or beans with nuts (think rice and beans or peanut butter and whole grain bread).

If vegetarian and vegan athletes are eating a well-balanced diet which contains a variety of these foods, they will be able to satisfy their protein and amino acid needs. However, it may be useful for these types of athletes to utilize protein bars and powders to supplement their diets.

Picking protein bars/powders (animal or plant-based):
- Check the ingredients. Look for red flags like "High Fructose Corn Syrup" and "Aspartame." Also, look for products with as few ingredients as possible. Many companies have come under scrutiny lately because of the extra junk they add into their protein powders. Check the ingredients for words you can't pronounce or understand, and look them up to make an educated decision whether or not you want to put it in your body. I advise finding products with five ingredients or less. It is also best to choose an option that's organic.
- Take the grams of protein per serving listed on the supplement facts panel and divide it by the serving size (in grams). This will give you the percentage of protein in each serving. The percent per serving should be 70

percent or greater.
- Look for low carbohydrate and fat options under 5g of carbohydrates and 3g of fat. Adequate amounts of carbohydrates and fats are easily obtainable from the rest of your diet.

So, how much protein should you be getting? The answer is different for each person and their goals. Read through the general guidelines below, and fill in your specific goals in Week Three of your Transition Plan.

> **TRANSITION PLAN**
> *Week Three - Macronutrients*
> Estimate your target protein, carbohydrates, fats, and calories, and start noting how you feel as you adjust your food intake.

When trying to lose weight, maintain muscle in heavy competition, or build muscle, it is advised to eat 0.6g to 0.9g of protein per pound of body weight in order to preserve your muscle mass, especially if you are very active.

Some bodybuilders shoot for 1g per pound of body weight, but the official position of The International Society of Sports Nutrition is between 0.6g to 0.9g per pound of body weight.[10] It has also been shown in multiple studies that there is no difference in muscle synthesis above 0.9g per pound of body weight—which goes against the common belief that to build muscle, 1g of protein per pound of body weight is optimal.[11]

---

[10] Campbell et al., "International Society of Sports Nutrition position stand: protein and exercise." This is converted from their recommendation of 1.4 to 2g per kilogram of body weight.

[11] M.A. Tarnopolsky, "Evaluation of protein requirements for trained strength athletes"; P.W. Lemon, "Protein requirements and muscle mass/strength changes during intensive training in novice bodybuilders"; J.R. Hoffman, "Effect of protein intake on strength, body composition and endocrine changes in strength/power athletes."

The International Society of Sports Nutrition also advises that individuals engaging in endurance exercise target the lower end of this range (0.6-0.7g), individuals engaging in intermittent activities should be more toward the middle (0.7-0.8g), and those engaging in strength and power exercises should be at the upper end of this range (0.8-0.9g).

A common mistake in many low calorie diets is to reduce all macronutrients (carbohydrates, protein, and fat) equally for a calorie deficit, as it results in burning both muscle and fat for energy, rather than just fat.

When I first started trying to manage my food intake post-sport, I started using a food-tracking app on my phone. It asked me how much weight I wanted to lose, and how fast. Of course I wanted to lose weight as fast as possible, so I picked the greatest amount it would let me lose per week. The app then gave me a calorie goal of 1,200 calories per day. Perfect, I thought! You mean all I have to do is count calorie intake? So I continued the same unhealthy foods, just less of them. I lost a few pounds. But, after the first few weeks I couldn't understand why I wasn't losing weight any more, and why I was feeling foggy-headed, exhausted, and constantly getting sick.

What happens if you do not adjust your macronutrients to be low in carbohydrates and adequate in protein is that you end up burning muscle as part of weight loss, thereby damaging your metabolism. Muscles are the largest calorie burners in your body, even at rest—so if you burn muscle, then come off a diet, you no longer have the ability to burn as many calories as you did prior to starting. Therefore, it's much easier to gain more fat back, even if you are eating overall healthier than you were before—and let's be honest, the typical yo-yo cycle is that we diet until we get the weight off, and then go right back to eating the way we were prior. Then, we decide to go back on a low-calorie diet to get the weight off once more, and burn more muscle. It's a vicious cycle.

The unfortunate fact is **all calories are not created equal**. It means we can't use the excuse that just because food is edible, it's nourishment. Different macronutrients are metabolized differently, and serve different purposes. The quality of the food is indeed important, and a food's nutrient density truly makes a difference. We will get into more detail about this later in the section.

The main difference between the diet of a competitive athlete and post-sport athlete comes down to hanging the balance of macronutrients. As you will see, the competitive athlete needs more fuel, and therefore more food, to sustain their lifestyle. (I know, shocking.)

When maintaining weight, aim to ingest at least half your body weight in grams of protein per day.

The United States Department of Agriculture (USDA) recommends 46g of protein for all adult women, and 56g of protein for all adult males.[12] It should be noted that these requirements are for sedentary individuals. Those who are more active need more protein, which is why half your body weight in grams is a good target, as it allows for difference in size.

Additionally, it is important to think about how to spread out your protein intake throughout the day. Many of us are actually

[12] "Dietary Guidelines 2015-2020."

protein deficient for much of the day, with muscle synthesis at less than maximal levels. A large amount of protein eaten at dinner is mostly wasted because the body can't use it all at one time. More even distribution of protein throughout the day is linked to chronic disease prevention, preservation of lean body mass, and bone health. Best practices for even protein distribution throughout the day are as follows:

Breakfast
Eating protein at breakfast will keep you feeling full longer, and even reduce tendencies to snack later in the day. Those who skip protein at breakfast also tend to have lower levels of calcium, potassium, magnesium, phosphorus and zinc, vitamins A, E, B6, C, and folate.

Pre- and Post-workout
Eat a food high in protein 30-60 minutes before and after your workout. This will help preserve and build muscle both during and after exercise.

Lunch
If you know it will be awhile before you eat again or have dinner, having protein at lunch can help hold you over until your next meal. It will also help curb those afternoon cravings.

Dinner
Eating some protein at dinner will help you fill up before your longest fasting period (sleep). It will also help with muscle and tissue recovery and repair while you rest.

Now that you are starting to develop an understanding of how much protein to eat throughout the day, you are probably wondering how much protein different foods contain. While

I've included some example items, the best way to learn how much protein is in a specific piece of food is to track your food intake. It's easiest to use your food tracking app. You should already have an idea of how much protein you are already getting. This week, adjust as needed.

Protein Count in Various Foods

1 egg = 6g
7 oz 2% Fage yogurt = 20g
1 oz cheddar cheese = 7g
1 slice Killer Dave's 21 Grain Bread = 5g
1 cup cooked brown rice = 5g
¼ cup dry steel cut oats = 7g
½ cup dry rolled oats = 7g
1 cup cooked quinoa = 8g
1 cup cooked black beans = 15g
3 oz tofu = 6g
1 cup edamame = 17g
1 oz raw peanuts = 7g
1 cup raw kale = 2g
1 cup spinach = 1g
1 oz chia seeds = 4g
1 oz sunflower seeds = 6g
3 oz chicken breast: 30g
3 oz chicken drumstick: 23g
3 oz chicken thigh: 31g
3 oz turkey breast: 15g
3 oz ground beef: 22g
3 oz brisket: 15g
3 oz corned beef: 15g
3 oz shoulder steak: 24g
3 oz tenderloin: 18g

3 oz ham: 19g
3 oz pork chop: 22g
3 oz pulled pork: 33g
3 oz lamb: 21g

Try not to get in a rut of eating the same type of protein every day, like chicken at every meal. Switch it up! The more you experiment, the more you will know what feels better for your body. Keep in mind that animal protein can also have saturated fat and cholesterol and, depending on where it came from, hormones, antibiotics, and e-coli. Unlike plant-based proteins, it also lacks phytonutrients, water, antioxidants, enzymes, and fiber—so it is wise to still include plant-based proteins in your diet to make sure you are getting these protective compounds.

Note that how an animal is cared for from birth to slaughter really does affect your body. The unsanitary (and inhumane) practices of factory farms are threatening our food supply. We are at the very top of the food chain, so when we consume an animal, we consume what those animals have eaten, any antibiotics the animal was given, and so on. The healthiest way to go about adding animal proteins in your diet is to eat organic, free range, and naturally fed. Look for the Certified Humane Seal, which is the gold standard in farming.

Carbohydrates

Carbohydrates are a main source of energy, and imperative for the brain and body to function properly. To understand the role of carbohydrates as a macronutrient, it's important that we first understand the basics of how we use food for energy.

The body has our means of fuel: glucose (carbohydrates), fatty acids (fats), amino acids (protein), and fat stores.

One of our body's survival mechanisms is to not give up its fat stores. This dates back to when we were hunters and gatherers, and we needed to preserve every bit of extra energy for survival. Such people were constantly moving to find food, build shelter, hunt, and run away from predators. They also needed every extra bit of stored energy for the winter when food was scarce. Unfortunately, we haven't evolved past this survival mechanism, and as you know, we no longer have the constant threat of a famine or saber-toothed tiger chasing us down.

The first energy source the body wants to use is glucose, or sugar from the broken down carbohydrates that it has digested. Your blood sugar rises when you eat carbohydrates, and must be brought back down. Specifically, the pancreas secretes insulin (a master hormone) to deal with the sugar by either taking it to muscles that need it for energy, or to the brain. But, what happens if we don't need all that energy? Insulin will then store that excess glucose as fat for later use.

Because athletes are expending so much energy, they need carbohydrates to support their activity (the amount depending on the sport). Having a sufficient amount of carbohydrates improves athletic performance by delaying fatigue and allowing an athlete to compete at higher levels for longer. However, if we are no longer as active as we were, we do not need as many carbohydrates to be sufficiently fueled. Therefore, the extra carbohydrates our body no longer needs is stored as fat for later use.

The less active you are, the less carbohydrates you burn. According to expert Mark Sisson, author of The Primal Blueprint and founder of Primal Nutrition, Inc., as well as what I've observed with my clients, below are carbohydrate ranges given for the typical body[13]. Note that this is not counting fiber, which does not affect blood sugar (subtract fiber from the total amount of carbohydrates to get the "net carb" count).

0-50g per day	nutritional ketosis (burning solely fat for energy)
50-100g per day	weight loss
100-150g per day	weight maintenance
150-300g per day	insidious weight gain
300g+ per day	danger zone for obesity and chronic disease

For many post-sport athletes, 100-150g of carbohydrates per day will work great for weight maintenance. However, some are more sensitive to carbohydrates and store fat more easily, and may need to reduce their carbohydrate intake to 50-100g per day to maintain weight. This is the case for those who are insulin resistant, which is when your body does not use insulin effectively, and blood sugar builds up in the blood instead of being absorbed by cells for energy (leading to Type II Diabetes). This may also be true for women as they go through menopause, as well as the elderly. The amount of carbohydrates one can tolerate can also be increased by continued exercise and strength training, which increases insulin sensitivity and overall metabolism. Adjust your current carbohydrate intake to meet your goals in your Transition Plan.

---

[13] "Dietary Guidelines 2015-2020."

However, the type of carbohydrates ingested is also a large factor. Like calories, not all carbohydrates are created equal.

Simple Versus Complex

There are two categories of carbohydrates: simple and complex. Complex carbohydrates are whole foods, as they still have all the fiber and protein contained within them. Simple carbohydrates consist of only one or two sugars and have had protein and fiber stripped from them through processing. Examples include refined sugar, white bread, white pasta, white rice, and processed foods. Because the fiber and proteins have been stripped from the molecule, they are more easily digested, and therefore hit our bloodstream much faster.

The faster carbohydrates enter the bloodstream, the more glucose insulin must distribute throughout the body as energy to bring blood sugar back down. If you aren't as active as before, your body may not need as much energy, and what remains will therefore be stored as fat.

Common Simple Carbohydrates

Sweeteners	sugar, syrups
White Grains and Pasta	white rice, white bread, white pasta, cereal, pastries
Snacks	chips, cookies, candy, cake, pretzels, soda, fruit juice, pie

Common Complex Carbohydrates

Dairy	2% or 4% yogurt, regular milk

Legumes	lentils, kidney beans, chick peas, split peas, soy beans, pinto beans
Whole Grain Bread and Pasta	buckwheat, brown rice, corn, wheat, barley, oats, sorghum, quinoa
Fruit and Vegetables	tomatoes, onions, cucumbers, dill pickles, carrots, yams, strawberries, peas, radishes, beans, broccoli, spinach, green beans, zucchini, apples, pears, cucumbers, asparagus, grapefruit, prunes, etc.

Athletes can make use of simple carbohydrates, as they may need quick-digesting sugars in sports that use bursts of energy, like basketball, soccer, or football. However, regardless of who you are, a best practice is to stick with complex carbohydrates. They take longer for your body to digest, and cause sugar to enter the bloodstream at a slower rate. Insulin can therefore direct the blood sugar as it comes in for energy use, resulting in less opportunity for it to be stored.

In short, this translates to cutting out processed foods and sugar. What's processed? Pretty much anything that comes in a package and has a nutrition label.

The Glycemic Index

Another guide to help you make the best decision about which carbs to eat is the Glycemic Index. The Glycemic Index tells you how quickly a food will digest, and therefore how it will affect your blood sugar. Foods are scored from 1-100, with sugar being 100. Those lower on the glycemic index are healthier for your body, and you will tend to feel full longer after eating them. The smaller the number, the less impact the food has on your blood sugar: 55 or less is low (good), 56-69 is medium, and 70 or higher is high (bad). Most complex carbs fall into the low glycemic index category. Some good examples can be seen below:

Type of Food	Poor Choice	Better Choice
Breakfast cereal	corn flakes (93)	oatmeal (55) 100% bran cereal (38)
Rice	white rice (64)	brown rice (50)
Bread	white bread (100) whole wheat (71)	whole grain bread (51)
Starch	baked potato without skin (98) French fries (75)	baked potato with skin (69) boiled sweet potato (44)
Pasta	white pasta, boiled (58)	whole grain pasta, boiled (42)

You can find additional ratings for other common foods at glycemicindex.com.

Fat

Fat has developed a bad reputation. In the 1950s, influential scientist Ancel Keys conducted his Seven Countries Study, comparing the health and diet of nearly 13,000 middle-aged men in the U.S., Japan, and Europe.[14] He found a correlation between people who ate greater amounts of animal protein (meat and

---

[14] "Time Magazine: We Were Wrong About Saturated Fats."

dairy) and heart disease than those who did not, concluding that saturated fat should be avoided. However, his research did not include data from nations that did not fit the hypothesis. And, within the data he published, populations existed in which diet and heart disease were far from his model. Despite these findings, Keys relentlessly advocated the theory that fat caused heart disease, persuading the American Heart Association (AHA) to issue the country's first-ever guidelines targeting saturated fat.[14]

The federal government went to the extreme of stating that all fat is unhealthy, and thereby began recommending a low-fat diet to the nation. Food companies began releasing low-fat or non-fat products to satisfy the masses. However, removing fat from a product means you remove much of the taste. And, what do you add when something doesn't taste good? Sugar.

Consider what you just learned about how simple carbohydrates negatively affect the body. Now, pair it with the fact that people gorge themselves on fat-free products while thinking they are eating healthy food. You just landed on the recipe for the obesity epidemic. Of course, our country's fat aversion isn't the only cause, but it's a huge mistake and a large contributor to the state we are in today.

The truth is fats are actually a very important part of a healthy diet. In fact, some fats even reduce the risk of heart disease.[15] They provide essential fatty acids, promote skin health, absorb vitamins and minerals, build cell membranes, aid in blood clotting, improve muscle movement, and help decrease inflammation. Fats are also another source of energy for longer duration and more intense activity. A lack of fat will prevent important hormones (such as steroid hormones that control how the body responds to

---

[15] "Omega-3 fatty acids."

high energy demands, maintain mineral balance, and drive muscle growth) from being in balance, and impair athletic performance. Although fats are important, it's still easy to get confused about which fats are good, which we should avoid, and how much fat we should eat. At a minimum, we need about 10 percent of our calories to come from fat, and the AHA recommends that fat should make up 20 to 35 percent of our food intake.[16] While most Americans get 34 percent or more, they are often not the healthy kind. The below points should help clear up common points of confusion.

Unsaturated, Saturated, and Trans Fats

Fat can be broken down into two groups: unsaturated and saturated.

Unsaturated Fats

Unsaturated fats fall into two categories—mono-unsaturated and polyunsaturated—and are most commonly found in plant-based foods and oils. When eaten in moderation, these fats can reduce "bad" LDL cholesterol levels and risk of heart disease.

Mono-unsaturated fats are a good source of the antioxidant vitamin E. Polyunsaturated fats help lower both blood cholesterol and triglyceride levels. Omega-3s are also found in polyunsaturated fats, and come from sources such as fatty fish, flaxseed, and walnuts. Omega-3 fatty acids are especially important in regulating inflammation. However, in the typical American diet, most of us are not getting anywhere near the recommended amount.[14] Most omega-3 experts recommend that adults should consume about 500 mg of omega-3 EPA/DHA

---

[16] "Know Your Fats."

per day (equivalent to two fatty fish meals per week) to maintain overall good health.[14] A diet low in omega-3 fatty acids can impair exercise recovery, cause fatigue, poor circulation, dry skin, poor memory, and mood swings or depression.

Mono-unsaturated Fat	Polyunsaturated Fat
Oils - olive, canola, sunflower, peanut, sesame	Oils - soybean, corn, safflower
Fruits - avocados, olives	Soy - milk, tofu
Nuts - almonds, peanuts, macadamia, hazelnuts, pecans, cashews	Seeds - sunflower, sesame, flax seed, pumpkin seeds
Nut butters - peanut, almond, cashew	Fatty fish - salmon, tuna, mackerel, herring, trout, sardines

Saturated Fats

There are two types of fat that should be eaten more sparingly: saturated and trans fatty acids. Both can raise cholesterol, clog arteries, and increase risk of heart disease—the leading cause of death in the United States. Saturated fats are found in animal products and in vegetable fats, such as coconut and palm oils.

There are two types of trans fats: those that are naturally occurring, such as those found in small amounts of dairy and meat; and artificial trans fats, which can occur when liquid oils are hardened into "partially-hydrogenated" fats to prevent a food from becoming rancid on the shelf. On a food label, you will see this listed as "partially hydrogenated oil." Natural trans fats are not a concern if eaten in moderation. The real worry is the artificial trans fats used in frying, baked goods, cookies, icings, crackers, packaged snack foods, microwave popcorn, and some margarines.

THE ATHLETE AFTER

In 2015, the FDA ruled that trans fat is not "generally recognized as safe," and gave food manufacturers three years to remove partially hydrogenated oils from their products. Some cities, like New York City and Philadelphia, have already banned their usage.[17]

Moderate Saturated / Natural Trans Fat (OK in Moderation)	Artificial Trans Fat (AVOID)
High-fat cuts of meat - beef, lamb, pork, chicken with skin	Commercially-baked foods - pastries, cookies, doughnuts, muffins, cakes
Whole-fat dairy - milk, cream, cheese, yogurt, butter	Packaged food - crackers, microwave popcorn, chips, candy bars
Oils - coconut, palm	Fried foods - French fries, fried chicken, chicken nuggets, breaded fish

Probably the most common question I receive regarding saturated fats is what type of dairy to choose: whole, 4 percent, 2 percent, skim, fat free… there are so many options! Depending on how you personally feel after eating dairy (many may find that they feel better the less they have), I recommend having the full-fat versions. This is because many companies will add sugar when they take fat out. If less fat is easier on your system, check your favorite brands to make sure they aren't adding sugar to their low-fat products compared to their full-fat counterparts.

---

[17] J. Christensen, "FDA orders food manufacturers to stop using trans fat within three years."

The best way to keep on top of the fats in your diet is to become a label reader. Look for foods that are low in saturated and trans fats. Bear in mind that a product with a label boasting "trans-fat free" can actually have up to 0.5 grams of trans fats per serving—and these can add up quickly.

By now, you may be wondering if there is a specific amount of fat you should aim for, as we discussed with protein and carbohydrates. The American Heart Association recommends that 20-35 percent of your total daily calories come from fat.[18] That's a large range. Here is a breakdown based on how we metabolize fat for energy:

< 20% calories from fat	risk increases for inadequate intakes of vitamin E and adverse changes in HDL cholesterol and triglycerides
20-25% calories from fat	low fat diet (good for people who struggle with heart disease, high cholesterol, trying to lose weight, etc.)
25-30% calories from fat	recommended for strength/power athletes (training at high intensity in short bursts) [19]
30-35% calories from fat	recommended for endurance athletes (training at a lower intensity for long periods of time) [20]
> 35% calories from fat	increases risk of obesity and heart disease

---

[18] K. Zerasky. "To track how much fat I eat each day"

[19] Scheet, Stoppani, and McGuigan, Michael. "NSCA Sports Nutrition Education Program."

[20] "Fat Intake for Endurance Athletes."

How Our Bodies Use Food for Energy

The body takes carbohydrates, fat, and protein to convert enough energy to adenosine triphosphate (ATP)—which is the fuel used in the cell. [21] There are two types of metabolisms your body can use: anaerobic and aerobic.

Anaerobic Metabolism

When oxygen can't get to the cells fast enough to create adequate energy to meet muscular demand, carbohydrates (glucose) are the only source that can be converted to ATP. Therefore, carbohydrates provide the main fuel used during high intensity exercise (like sprinting and lifting heavy weights).

Aerobic Metabolism

When there is enough oxygen available to meet the demand of the muscles, carbohydrates fatty acids, amino acids from protein, and fat stores can be converted to ATP. Therefore, endurance athletes should take in higher amounts of fatty acids in their macronutrient balance.

Protein can also be utilized to create ATP, but the key structural role and multiple other functions of amino acids make it an important nutrient to spare, so it is used when there is not enough carbohydrates or fatty acids available. This is why it's important to get enough protein, so that there is enough available to support muscle and it does not get broken down for energy. Fat stores are the final tank tapped, as our body wants to hold on to these reserves for survival.

---

[21] Wendy Bumgardner. "Anaerobic Metabolism vs. Aerobic Metabolism."

Your body will often switch between aerobic and anaerobic metabolisms during sports and exercise activities that require short bursts of sprints as well as sustained jogging, such as soccer, tennis, and basketball. [21]

Have you ever been on a cardio machine at the gym and seen the heart rate zone chart that shows the range for the fat burning zone, aerobic zone, anaerobic zone, etc.? This shows where your heart rate should be depending on your goals. Is your goal to burn fat? Gain more endurance? The faster your heart rate, the harder your body is working to get oxygen to the cells and create energy to keep up. Simply going on a brisk walk may be what you need to burn fat (if that's your goal, of course).

> **TRANSITION PLAN**
> *Week Four - Food Adjustment*
> Now that you have been more conscious of how much protein, carbohydrates, fats, and calories to be aiming for, continue adjusting your diet based on your goals and how you feel.

To get a general idea of your maximum heart rate, subtract your age from 220. The below chart shows the benefits of exercising within a certain heart rate zone, based on your maximum heart rate.

50-60%	Very light exercise: helps with recovery
60-70%	Light exercise: improves basic endurance and fat burning
70-80%	Moderate exercise: improves aerobic fitness
80-90%	Hard exercise: increases maximum performance capacity
90-100%	Maximum: helps athletes develop maximum speed and performance

Overall Calorie Intake

I mentioned earlier that it is often more helpful to focus on the type of calories you eat, rather than on caloric intake, since all calories aren't created equal. Now that you have your macronutrient goals, you can figure out your calorie range from there. For a step-by-step guide on how to do this, turn to your Transition Plan.

Micronutrients and Nutrient Density

So far, we've been over the macronutrients that give us calories: protein, carbohydrates, and fat. But what those macronutrients are made up of is equally, if not more, important. Micronutrients are the non-caloric food factors, such as vitamins, minerals, fibers, and phytochemicals.[22] The key to optimizing health and achieving the ideal body weight is for the majority of food intake to have a relatively high proportion of nutrients to calories.[22]

> **TRANSITION PLAN**
> *Week Five - Micronutrients*
> Focus on fitting in these healthy superfoods to make sure you are getting the nutrients you need every day.

Remember, although you may have an idea of how many calories to consume, it isn't always about how many calories you eat, but rather what kind. Just because a label lists the number of calories a food contains, it doesn't mean they will be digested or absorbed equally. Labels can also be incorrect about how many calories are in a food. Companies are allowed a 20 percent margin of error!

---

[22] "Nutrient Density."

This is why it's better to think of a food's nutrient density, rather than its caloric density. I like using Dr. Joel Fuhrman's acronym G-BOMBS to remember what the most nutrient-dense foods are on the planet. Dr. Fuhrman, health and fitness enthusiast, board-certified family physician, and New York Times best-selling author and nutritional researcher, has described that these foods should make up a significant portion of your diet.[22]

"G" is for Greens

Raw, leafy greens contain only about 100 calories per pound and can be consumed in unlimited quantities. The majority of calories in green vegetables, including leafy greens, come from protein. This plant protein is also packaged with beneficial phytochemicals: folate (the natural form of folic acid), calcium, and small amounts of omega-3 fatty acids. Leafy greens are also rich in antioxidant pigments called carotenoids, which are known to promote healthy vision, and contain substances that protect blood vessels and are associated with reduced risk of diabetes.

Some examples of leafy greens are bok choy, broccoli, and kale. These are all part of the cruciferous vegetable family, which have a unique chemical composition with a variety of potent anti-cancer effects. Isothiocyanates (ITCs) also work to remove carcinogens, reduce inflammation, neutralize oxidative stress, inhibit angiogenesis (the process by which tumors acquire a blood supply), and kill cancer cells.

Some ways I incorporate leafy greens into my diet that go beyond salads are by adding them to smoothies (with berries—another superfood) and incorporating them in main dishes, such as putting sautéed kale on homemade pizza or in stews.

"B" is for Beans

Beans (and other legumes as well) are the most nutrient-dense carbohydrate source. They act as an anti-diabetes and weight-loss food because they are digested slowly and have a stabilizing effect on blood sugar, which helps to prevent food cravings. Plus, they contain soluble fiber, which lowers cholesterol levels.

Beans are also unique because they have very high levels of fiber and resistant starch. They not only help reduce the total number of calories absorbed from beans, but they are also fermented by intestinal bacteria into fatty acids that help prevent colon cancer. Eating beans, peas, or lentils at least twice a week has been found to decrease colon cancer risk by 50 percent. Legume intake also provides significant protection against oral, larynx, pharynx, stomach, and kidney cancers. Add them to your burritos, make some delicious chili, or even make your own black bean burger patties.

"O" is for Onions

Onions, along with leeks, garlic, chives, shallots, and scallions, make up the Allium family of vegetables. They have beneficial effects on the cardiovascular and immune systems, as well as anti-diabetic and anti-cancer effects. Similar to the ITCs in cruciferous vegetables, Alliums contain organosulfur compounds, which are released when onions are chopped, crushed, or chewed. Epidemiological studies have found that increased consumption of Allium vegetables is associated with lower risk of gastric and prostate cancers due to these compounds.[22] They prevent the development of cancers by detoxifying carcinogens, halting cancer cell growth, and blocking angiogenesis. Onions also contain quercetin, which slows tumor development, suppresses growth and proliferation, and induces cell death in colon cancer cells. Flavonoids, compounds found in plants that serve antioxidant benefits, also have anti-inflammatory effects that may contribute to cancer prevention. Try adding red onions on top of your salad, in burritos or tacos, or in omelets.

"M" is for Mushrooms

Consuming mushrooms regularly can help decrease risk of breast, stomach, and colorectal cancers. Dr. Fuhrman references one recent Chinese study, in which women who ate at least 10 grams of fresh mushrooms each day (about one mushroom per day) had a 64 percent decreased risk of breast cancer.[22] Even more dramatic protection was gained by women who ate 10 grams of mushrooms and drank green tea daily—an 89 percent decrease in breast cancer risk for premenopausal women, and an 82 percent decrease for postmenopausal women, respectively. White, cremini, Portobello, oyster, shiitake, maitake, and reishi mushrooms all have anti-cancer properties—some are anti-inflammatory, stimulate the immune system, prevent DNA damage, slow cancer cell growth, cause programmed cancer cell death, and inhibit angiogenesis. Add mushrooms to omelets, salads, stir-fry, and one of my favorites—quiche.

"B" is for Berries

Blueberries, strawberries, and blackberries are true super foods, containing more antioxidants than any other food on the planet. Although naturally sweet and juicy, berries are low in sugar and high in nutrients and therefore among the best foods you can eat. Their antioxidant content produces both cardio-protective and anti-cancer effects, such as reducing blood pressure and inflammation, preventing DNA damage, inhibiting tumor angiogenesis, and stimulating the body's own antioxidant enzymes. Berry consumption has been linked to reduced risk of diabetes, cancers, and cognitive decline. Berries are also an excellent food for the brain, as consumption improves both motor coordination and memory. My favorite way to add berries to my diet is at breakfast, either in a smoothie or with yogurt.

"S" is for Seeds

Seeds and nuts contain healthy fats and are rich in a spectrum of micronutrients, including phytosterols, minerals, and antioxidants. Countless studies have demonstrated their cardiovascular benefits and how including nuts in your diet aids in weight maintenance and diabetes prevention.

Seeds are also abundant in trace minerals and are higher in protein than nuts. Flax, chia, and hemp seeds are extremely rich sources of omega-3 fats. In addition to the omega-3s, flaxseeds are rich in fiber and lignans. Flaxseed and sesame seed consumption protects against heart disease through a number of different mechanisms, and lignans have anti-cancer effects. Sunflower seeds are especially rich in protein and minerals. Pumpkin seeds are rich in iron and calcium, and are a good source of zinc. Sesame seeds have the greatest amount of calcium of any food in the world, and provide abundant amounts of vitamin E. Also, black sesame seeds are extremely rich in antioxidants. The healthy fats in seeds and nuts also aid in the absorption of nutrients when eaten with vegetables. I incorporate seeds and nuts by throwing them on my salad. I also add flaxseed to smoothies, and eat handfuls of nuts as a snack.

If you want to learn more about G-BOMBS, check out Dr. Fuhrman's book *Super Immunity: The Essential Nutrition Guide for Boosting Your Body's Defenses to Live Longer, Stronger, and Disease Free.*

Katie Hargrave

Nutrition and the Mind

Integrated within this section are topics that address how different foods affect the body. But, what's only briefly touched on is how nutrition affects the mind. Having a balance of the right protein, carbohydrate, fat, and micronutrients is important for your body and mind to function at its best. Can you function without the right proportions? Yes. Will you be at your best performance level? No. This is why the right nutritional stasis is so important for us all, competing or not. Maintaining your ideal weight doesn't necessarily mean you are functioning at your best—and isn't that what we all want, during sports and beyond?

Balanced nutrition can positively affect the mind. Having the right amino acids in protein intake is important for focus, dealing with stress, mental clarity, memory, and overall brain function. Achieving the right amounts of omega-3 to omega-6 fatty acids is crucial for memory and cognitive performance. The brain uses half of the glucose (blood sugar from carbohydrates) in the body, making complex carbohydrates crucial for thinking, memory, and learning.[23] However, as with anything in nutrition, too much can be a bad thing. High levels of blood glucose can affect the brain's functional connectivity, or how it links different regions of its functional properties together.[17] Too much sugar can also literally cause the brain to atrophy and shrink.[17] Therefore, a balance in blood sugar is not only essential to maintain a healthy weight, but also to maintain healthy brain function.

---

[23] "Sugar and the Brain."

Putting it all Together

By now, you have hopefully started tracking your food intake, calculated and adjusted for your macronutrients, and begun experimenting with different foods and how they make you feel. The key is to get into a habit of cooking whole foods, rather than easy and quick-to-prepare processed foods.

Meal planning is also important to prevent coming home from a long, exhausting day at work to no dinner, resulting in ordering out or making something quick and unhealthy. For a free sample meal-prep plan, visit my website at athleteafterword.com.

Continue to track your food and note how you feel for as long as you need. Note what you learned about yourself on your Transition Plan, and share with me and the athlete community at facebook.com/athleteafter.

BODY

THE ATHLETE AFTER

Post-Sport Exercise

The post-sport athlete usually does one of two things when they retire: continue training at their competition volume, failing to realize they can be healthy with reduced exercise intensity; or, stop training all together because they are exhausted from a life of exercise and believe they deserve a break.

Let's start with the first situation. You've been training for years to be the best at your specific sport and position. This could mean that for a defensive tackle, you've been scarfing down as much food as possible and lifting extremely heavy for a long time in order to be big and strong enough for your position. Or, it could mean that as a cross-country runner, you've been putting in 70-plus miles per week and eating more fat than carbohydrates. Post-competition, it isn't realistic or healthy for the football player to continue carrying as much excess weight (let's be real—it isn't all muscle). And, although the runner may continue logging miles, new career and life goals may make previous distance runs unrealistic to maintain. Once you refocus on a new career, or perhaps start a family, or both—there may simply no longer be enough hours in the day to continue training at the rate at which you have been accustomed.

There is also such a thing as exercising too much.

Excess Exercise: Stress and the Body

Our autonomic nervous system (ANS) is responsible for the

involuntary functions of the body, or the functions that happen automatically without our having to think about them (heart beating, digestion, etc.). The ANS is comprised of the parasympathetic nervous system (PNS) and sympathetic nervous system (SNS). Depending on the situation, one of these systems is dominant at any given time.

The parasympathetic nervous system controls homeostasis (physiological equilibrium) and is responsible for the body's "rest and digest" function. Its nerves stimulate digestion, as well as the immune and eliminative organs. These organs include the liver, pancreas, stomach, and intestines. Moving yourself into a healthy parasympathetic state where the body can regenerate and eliminate toxins—and staying there as much of the time as possible—helps heal health conditions, aid in muscle recovery, losing weight, and detoxing the body.

The sympathetic nervous system controls the body's responses to a perceived threat and is responsible for the "fight or flight" response. Think back to when humans were hunters and gatherers, and why it was important to have this capability: in case we were without food or being hunted. For this reason, our body holds on to stored energy (fat) in case it needs to survive without food or will need emergency energy to escape. The "fight or flight" response also prevents us from sleeping deeply, because we are on high alert to be able to wake up and react quickly. Our body is able to focus on these survival mechanisms by moving away from "unnecessary" organ functions like digestion, elimination, and healing. Instead, it puts all its efforts into critical functions, such as increasing blood circulation, which causes blood pressure to rise. Insulin begins to convert glycogen (stored emergency energy within muscle) into glucose for the body to use. Ever wonder how people are able to muster up crazy amounts of energy in an emergency situation? This is how.

Exercising for long periods of time at a high intensity is interpreted by the body as stress, which initiates the SNS. Your body doesn't know the difference between running a marathon and running away from a predator. If excess exercise keeps our bodies in the SNS zone, as described above, we actually hold onto fat as a survival mechanism.

Nutritional Biochemist Dr. Libby Weaver illustrates the excess exercise trap well. She mentioned in a lecture that she would run five to 10 miles almost every day as part of her workout routine. One summer she was hired to work at a retreat center where she started incorporating Tai Chi, causing her to cut back on running. She was amazed to find she lost weight during that summer, even though she wasn't getting nearly as much cardio. The reason for this outcome is she kept her body in the PNS, where her body was less stressed. Her body was therefore able to release stored fat because it knew it wasn't needed.

Incorporating mind-body exercise into your routine, among other benefits, can aid in getting your body into the PNS. Mind-body exercise is a physical activity performed with a meditative or sensory-awareness component.[24] It is executed with inward mental focus and special attention to breathing, which is beneficial in managing stress, deterioration of musculoskeletal health, decreased balance, high blood pressure, depression, pain, and decreased self-confidence.[24] Some examples of mind-body exercise include yoga, tai chi, qigong, pilates, tae kwon do, karate, and meditative walking.

---

[24] Ralph La Forge, "Mind-Body Exercise."

Katie Hargrave

How Much Exercise in Enough?

Now, let's discuss the second situation for those (like me) who decide to go on a gym hiatus. Typically, we make an excuse for a break thinking the way we have been exercising is the way we must continue—and, the thought is exhausting. However, doing something is always better than doing nothing. You may not think that getting out for a 10-minute walk with your dog is even worth it—but remember what we learned about aerobic exercise and fat burning? And, your dog will appreciate it, too. Don't tell yourself that just because you don't have two hours to spend at the gym, that it's not worth going. You can get in a good sweat in even just 15 minutes. In the past I've even had clients who have seen results in as little as one 30-minute session per week!

> **TRANSITION PLAN**
> *Week Six - Physical Activity*
> Make a commitment now to incorporate exercise into your week.

But, what should you aim for? An unnerving statistic is that after age 25, adults will lose about five pounds of muscle per decade without strength training.[25] Muscles are our biggest calorie burner! The more we have, the more calories we burn, and the more we can eat (and I know that is something that we all resonate with). Although exercise will vary by individual, the American Heart Association recommends[26]:

- 150 minutes of moderate physical activity per week (30 minutes, five days per week), or 25 minutes of intense

---

[25] Wayne Westcott, "Resistance Training."

[26] "American Heart Association Recommendation for Physical Activity in Adults."

activity three days per week for a total of 75 minutes.

- Moderate- to high-intensity muscle strengthening activity at least two days per week.

As athletes, we are competitive and typically want to push ourselves hard. That's what we've been trained to do, after all. However, what tends to happen when we push really hard post sport is we become exhausted. Since we no longer have a coach forcing us to continue or help regulate recovery, many of us exhaust or injure ourselves, then we stop or pull back too much. And, the cycle repeats. As a result, it's better to exercise moderately at a level you can maintain, even if that means going to the gym or walking one to two times per week, playing on a city league team one night per week, or fitting in a yoga class. You have to identify what works best for your lifestyle and then set goals.

For example, perhaps your position required you to be strong and powerful, and now you want to lean out. Or, maybe your joints are sore from years of pounding on the pavement or court, and you want to maintain your cardio with alternative activities. I highly recommend that if you have specific goals in mind that you talk to a personal trainer (and if you are in the Olympia/Tumwater area, I can help you with that!).

The key is to continue to make goals. Without knowing where you want to be, you aren't going to get there. Whether it is to finish your first bicycle tour, run a mile, or do 20 push-ups, list out your goals. When you reach them, make new ones. For us athletes, that's how we keep motivated. There needs to be an element of fun, achievement, and a feeling of progression.

Katie Hargrave

What Type of Athlete Are You?

Alan Couzens, exercise physiologist and Ironman coach, believes all of us are born with different mental wiring that affects how we respond to a given stimulus.[27] I believe this may be why some people are constantly seeking to push their bodies to the limit (cyclists who participate in the Race Across America, mountaineers who climb the Seven Summits, Ironman participants, etc.), and why others think those thrill-seekers are crazy. On a much smaller scale, I think this mental wiring is part of what separates the athletes from the non-athletes—those willing to push themselves through pain, give up so much of their lives, all for satisfaction of what they have been able, or are able, to accomplish.

According to Couzens, on one end or the spectrum you have "high reactives," those who perceive any given stimulus as more intense than average (for example, this may include introverts who find high stimuli environments very taxing, or those who need frequent period of quiet and solitude to recharge). On the other end of the spectrum, you have "low reactives," or those who need to actively seek stimuli to feel happy. These people are the skydivers, those who are extremely social, etc. For a post-sport athlete, this may result in the high-reactives hiding at home to relax, where the low reactives need exercise for their satisfaction.

It is thought that where an individual lies along the scale of high and low reactives depends on their hormones/neurotransmitters: dopamine and serotonin. Dopamine is a

---

[27] Alan Couzens, "What Type of Athlete Are You?"

natural "upper" that amplifies experiences and makes the individual more aware of his/her environment. It makes sense then that individuals with above-normal levels of this neurotransmitter would be motivated to "quiet things down," while those with low levels would be on the look out to "amp things up." Serotonin is the "sleepy/happy" neurotransmitter. For high reactive, stressed out types, serotonin helps quiet down some of the sensitivity to outside stimuli. So, while the low reactives are out hunting for dopamine, the high reactives are searching for serotonin. Fortunately, exercise (of the right type) can give both types exactly what they need.

Studies have shown there is a difference in dopamine and serotonin response depending on the intensity and duration of exercise.[27] High intensity, short duration exercise releases high levels of dopamine and serotonin. However, as intensity is reduced and duration is increased, dopamine falls below resting levels, and serotonin increases. High serotonin and low dopamine levels can lead to that "happy" state for high reactives (for example, "runners high"). If you are a low reactive participating in longer duration exercise at low intensity, you may notice that haven't experienced this sensation.

This information about yourself is important because it will determine which type of exercise plan is best for you. Will a sensation-seeking athlete stick with a slow aerobic workout that leaves

> **TRANSITION PLAN**
> *Week Seven - Exercise Goals*
> Brainstorm what will motivate you to get moving, and set activity goals.

them feeling tired and run down? Or will an introvert thrive off high-intensity competitive group training?

Chart by Athletic Type Based on Dopamine and Serotonin Levels[23]

Volume →

High Reactive/Low Response Does well with high frequency, high volume, low intensity modes of activity	Low Reactive/Low Response Does well with varied stimuli of mixed intensity.
	Low Reactive/High Response Does well with short bouts of focused and intense work.

Intensity →

High Reactivity/Low Training Response
(High Dopamine/Low Serotonin)

This type of athlete is extra sensitive to environmental stimuli. They are typically more of a loner and enjoy predictable and monotonous training programs. While they may enjoy occasional competition, too much competition or competitive training situations may be very psychologically stressful. Try long duration, low intensity training such as long distance running, cycling, hiking, swimming, etc.

Low Reactivity/Low Training Response
(Low Dopamine/Low Serotonin)

This type of athlete is craving the sort of satisfaction that comes from good, solid, work. They rarely get sick or injured despite high workloads, and can get bored with too much routine. They are prime candidates for exercise addiction, and on the other end if the volume drops, it can leave him/her feeling empty and sometimes even depressed (and possibly at higher risk for weight gain). One of the greatest challenge is convincing them to take a break for recovery. Varied types of exercise are needed to keep them interested, such as some cardio, high intensity interval training (HIIT), team sports, different workout classes, yoga, outdoor sports, etc.

Low Reactivity/High Response
(Low Dopamine/High Serotonin)

These athletes crave competition and thrive in a competitive atmosphere, but must be careful of over-training. Too much low intensity aerobic work will make them tired and take from their natural speed and strength. Too much high intensity work will quickly break these athletes. For these athletes, it is a fine balance between doing enough to keep the fire lit while protecting them from training too hard. Competitive environments like organized races, triathlons, CrossFit, etc. keep this athlete training consistently and sense of satisfaction.

For the same reasons it's important for young athletes to play a variety of sports. Adding alternative forms of activity to what you've been accustomed to provides many benefits, including injury prevention, rehabilitation, increased overall fitness, motivation, and rejuvenation. This is an excellent opportunity to try new things you previously haven't had time for—or even go back to the activities that brought you so much joy as a child.

If you are interested in team sports:

Check with your local Parks and Recreation Department to see what organized adult leagues are available in your area. Some common sports include basketball, soccer, volleyball, flag football, softball, cycling, dodgeball, bowling, bocce ball, kickball, curling, and even mini golf.

If you are interested in solo events:

Check your city calendar to see what local events are available. Perhaps you can train toward a 5k, half-marathon, or marathon, depending on your experience and goals. Or, you may decide to try a triathlon or duathlon. Having an event to work toward is a great tool for motivation, and still provides a feeling of participation and accomplishment on which we athletes thrive!

Exercising with Chronic Issues

You may find that certain parts of your body may not like some of your chosen activities due to strain from years of one sport. Overuse or chronic injuries are commonly diagnosed and usually require a period of rest combined with therapy. They may need a longer time to heal than you would like, but most will resolve with little or no long-term problems. Note that water and healthy omega-3 filled fats can help speed along the healing process. Some natural supplementation can also help. For more details, see page 85.

Joints

If you have trouble with your joints, try incorporating non-weight bearing exercises, such as elliptical trainers, cross-country ski machines, stationary bikes, swimming, and water running. However, keep in mind that to keep your bones strong, you do need some weight bearing activity, such as walking, running, and jumping.

Tendonitis

If you have tendonitis, it's advisable to refrain from anything that will put stress on the affected portion of your body. If you have not already seen a doctor about this issue, I suggest you do so to obtain a referral to a physical therapist who can work on helping you recover by giving you specific strengthening exercises and stretching positions. If you are experiencing pain in your upper body, try running or cycling for your cardio. If you are experiencing pain in your legs, try getting your cardio from swimming or a rowing machine.

Tennis/Golfers Elbow

Again, it is best to pay a visit to your physician and/or physical therapist for specific treatment. In general, it is recommended to avoid "grippy workouts," such as pull-ups, farmer's carries, kettlebell swings, etc. When your pain is less than two out of 10, ease back into upper body workouts. In the meantime, focus on core work and cardio exercises like running, jumping, and stationary biking.

Stress Fractures

Commonly, stress fractures occur in the foot, and must be diagnosed and treated by an orthopedic surgeon. Stress fractures of the metatarsals are treated with modified weight bearing, casting, and, in some instances, surgery. Talk to your doctor about non-weight bearing exercises.

Katie Hargrave

Accepting Your Body

One of the most challenging things about the post-sport change in activity level can be the change in the body itself. What many of us experience once we enter the "real world" of full-time work, family, etc., is we don't have the same amount of time to dedicate to exercise. As a result, our bodies change. This is especially true if our diet doesn't change with us.

All of a sudden, things may get a little squishier and less defined. This was the original reason I started crash dieting and working out for hours and hours after I put on 20 pounds. For the first time, I didn't like my body. I never thought I would be that person, but there were times when I looked in the mirror and absolutely loathed myself. It wasn't until I started caring more about what was going on inside my body than out that I was able to overcome this mental barrier.

You have to love yourself enough and know that you are worth treating your body with only the best to make a true lifestyle change. That's a hard thing to do, and something I still struggle with sometimes, even now. There are days I look in the mirror and think negative judgments about myself that I would never think about anyone else. Then, I remind myself how thankful I am for what my body does, and how lucky I truly am:

- It has given me the ability to play a sport well enough to get a college scholarship.
- I am able to live nearly every day without pain.
- I have no major illness.
- I am able to have a job as a personal trainer.
- I am able to walk and run with my dogs.
- I can hug my family and friends, and hold my son.

THE ATHLETE AFTER

My list of appreciations could go on and on. I try to remind myself how much I have to be thankful for when those thoughts start creeping into my mind. In your Transition Plan, list the reasons you are thankful for what your body does for you.

If you are struggling with body image issues, go to a mirror right now and tell yourself that you are beautiful. Say it out loud. And, tell yourself that you love yourself. Do this every time you wake up in the morning and before you go to bed at night.

> **TRANSITION PLAN**
> *Week Eight - Self Love*
> Take time to complete the given exercises on self-love and appreciation.

You can also put a positive affirmation on your mirror, as the background of your phone, in your wallet—wherever you are going to see it and read it the most.

Every day, make a note of something different you love about yourself. You will start to realize that there is so much to love!

Make a board of positive and inspiring quotes. I made one on Pinterest, and whenever I started feeling bad about myself, I would read through these quotes to help me get my mind back on track.

Pretty soon, you won't have to tell yourself how beautiful you are and that you love yourself every time you look in the mirror because you will automatically think it. You won't need the positive affirmation you wrote because you will be living it. You won't need to write down something you love about yourself every day because you will start recognizing reasons you love yourself throughout the day. You won't need other quotes, because you yourself will be an inspiration.

Mind-Body Connection

As we move closer to our section dedicated to the mind, it is worth addressing the mind-body connection. A healthy brain starts with a healthy body. Your body and mind are connected by nerve bundles, which move muscles and keep your organs functioning. Sensory stimuli are provided to the brain through these nerves.

There is neurobiological support for how and why mind-body therapies such as meditation and mind-body exercise interact with cognitive functions of the brain.[24] Muscle afferent pathways carry sensory information from the muscles and joints to the brain, giving direct access of muscular activity to our perception and cognition.[24] Therefore, exercise physically changes your brain.

Many brain health programs begin by focusing on physical health. A quarter of the blood our heart circulates is dedicated to the brain. Therefore, the stronger your heart, the more efficient the brain. A healthy heart requires a balanced, nutritional diet low in saturated fat and high in fiber and antioxidants, as well as regular exercise.

It is important to understand the ways in which to stimulate our brains, and what substance (in addition to lack of exercise), can limit the flow of blood to the brain[28]:

- **Nicotine:** Smoking cuts the flow of blood to every organ.
- **Dehydration:** The brain is 80 percent water; without adequate hydration, it is difficult to perform physical acts and hard to focus.
- **Caffeine:** In addition to reducing blood flow, caffeine also disrupts sleep and causes dehydration (however, research also suggests that a small amount of coffee or tea each day may benefit the brain as a little caffeine can improve attention—essential to learning and memory).
- **Lack of Sleep:** Studies have shown that those who sleep less than six hours per night have decreased blood flow to the brain, which impairs memory, mood, and cognitive function (it also means you are more likely to gain weight).[28]
- **Drugs and Alcohol:** The toxic effect of these substances harm blood vessels. An exception is red wine, which contains the ingredient "resveratrol." In moderation, it actually protects blood vessels.
- **Diabetes:** This disease causes blood vessels to grow brittle, and prevents proper healing of damaged tissue. It also increases the risk of a stroke.
- **Stress:** When the body reacts to potential danger, real or imagined, the endocrine glands prepare us to fight against an enemy or predator, or prepare us to run away (putting us in the SNS "fight or flight" mode). The flood of stress hormone adrenaline slows blood to the muscles at the expense of other regions. A bit of stress can actually spark higher achievement, but chronic stress can damage the brain due to the change of blood flow. Spikes in pressure can leave blood vessels vulnerable to breaking, impair memory, and create difficulty concentrating and learning. It's worth noting that caffeine also puts us in the SNS—therefore too

---

[28] Michael Sweeney and Cynthia Green, "Complete Guide to Brain Health."

much caffeine can be detrimental in multiple ways.

So, if we eliminate (or at least reduce!) substances that decrease blood flow, and increase exercise, we are taking steps towards a healthier brain with a better capacity for concentration, memorization, learning, and function. Studies have found that even walking for just ten minutes a day can boost energy levels for an hour. Whatever elevates your pulse and gets you sweating improves the function of your heart and lungs.

Athletes have more than likely been focusing on athletic performance, perhaps without even realizing the affect physical activity has on the brain. When you decrease your activity level, you may notice your concentration is impaired. To counteract this effect, you may instead have found yourself reaching for a cup of coffee (or any other source of caffeine) in an attempt to find focus from a different source.

Lack of exercise can also affect mental well-being. Every day for years, athletes have received regular doses of serotonin, the "feel good" hormone/neurotransmitter. When this suddenly decreases or is stopped outright, there is actually an upset to the chemistry of the body. This means lack of exercise affects post-sport athletes even more than the average Joe. Another reason to keep moving!

MIND

Identity: I Am an Athlete

Whether you are an athlete who is currently competing, or are "retired," you will always think of yourself as an athlete. This is a key reason why I identify with those who have put their competition days behind them as post-sport athletes—it's almost offensive not to acknowledge the athlete in someone who has dedicated that much time and energy to their craft.

Everyone has their own idea about what they must achieve to identify themselves with a certain designation, such as a writer, an artist, an actor, etc.. Malcolm Gladwell wrote in his book *Outliers* that it takes 10,000 hours of deliberate practice to become an expert. Nike co-founder Bill Bowerman said that if you have a body, you're an athlete. I disagree: I think it's a badge you earn.

But, what can be dangerous is identifying yourself as an athlete above all else. When that becomes who you are, rather than what you do, the transition out of sports can prove difficult.

A measure of athletic identity was introduced in a 1993 study, and referred to as "the degree to which an individual identifies with the athlete role and looks to others for acknowledgment of that role."[29] If being an athlete is your dominant role, its loss may affect your overall self-concept. It can happen suddenly, and even unexpectedly. For athletes who are so immersed in their sport that they haven't put effort into other areas (academics, hobbies, or social circles), or for those whose athletic career is cut short by an injury, the conclusion can cause a full on identity crisis. Others may think that because

---

[29] B.W. Brewer, et al "Athletic Identity."

they have invested time in other activities and outside friends, they will do just fine in the transition (that was me). Such people often come to find out that it still isn't an easy change, no matter how prepared they think they are.

Changing Focus

Let's not kid ourselves that having athletic abilities in this country doesn't provide an elite status. Losing this status alone is a difficult change for many.

When an athlete transitions from his or her sport to a new focus, a typical desire is role or skillset acknowledgment. But, the game has changed. You have a finely developed and specific skillset, and sometimes channeling these skills into a new role can be especially challenging.

Let's say you played a team sport for many years, but now your job requires you to sit in a desk, barely interacting with your coworkers throughout the day. If teamwork is how you thrive, you may not be as successful as you could. Or, if you are extremely competitive, but there is no room to grow in your current job—where do you go next? Take the time to understand what has been driving you thus far, and channel it into a career that fits. Finding a focus that is the right fit for you is important not only to be successful, but also to fill the spot that your sport and/or team once held.

Reflect on what pushed you through grueling workouts, day after day, and year after year. Was it to make yourself better, driving you to be recognized as the very best at your craft? Was it to fit in, or to be accepted? Was it for a scholarship to attain an education? Focusing on your strengths gained from these experiences will help you understand how you can channel them into your next focus—whether career or hobby. This exercise will help you focus on the positives you've gained your athletics, rather than a loss of how you once identified yourself.

If you have trouble pinpointing your strengths, and need more support on how to align your personality traits to help you achieve more, I recommend taking Tony Robbin's 15-minute online DISC Profile assessment. Tony Robbins is an entrepreneur, best-selling author, philanthropist, and renowned life and business strategist. He has also served as an advisor to leaders around the world for more than 38 years.

Robbin's test helps you to understand behavioral styles and personality types, so you can identify and maximize personal strengths. The report includes:

- **The Elements of DISC**: educational background behind the profile, the science and the four dimensions of behavior.
- **The DISC Dimensions**: a closer look at each of your four behavioral dimensions.
- **Style Summary**: a comparison of your natural and adaptive behavioral styles.
- **Behavioral Strengths**: a detailed strengths-based description of your overall behavioral style.
- **Communication**: tips on how you like to communicate.
- **Ideal Job Climate**: your ideal work environment.
- **Effectiveness**: insights into how you can be more effective by understanding your behavior.
- **Behavioral Motivations**: ways to ensure your environment is motivational.

- **Continual Improvement:** areas where you can focus on improving.
- **Training & Learning Style**: your preferred means of sharing and receiving styles.
- **Relevance Section**: making the information real and pertinent to you.
- **Success Connection**: connecting your style to your own life.

Take the survey at tonyrobbins.com/ue/ and include your observations in your Transition Plan.

Once you know which direction is best for you and you start applying for jobs, remember to list your athletic achievements on your resume. Coming out of school, I thought I was a step behind others who didn't play a sport in college and instead were able to gain work experience, or at least secure internships. However, I later found out after I was hired by my first employer that the reason he hired me was because I had been a student athlete. He could tell I was great at time-management, was able to take criticism, would be a good team player, was a leader, and that I could strategize.

> **TRANSITION PLAN**
> *Week Nine - Channeling Your Skillset*
> Take the DISC survey and list your qualities to pinpoint what you need from your career to be successful.

The Journal of Leadership & Organizational Studies underscores the athlete advantage, noting that former student-athletes are believed to possess higher levels of leadership, confidence, and self-esteem.[30] Numerous studies

---

[30] Kevin M. Kniffin, Brian Wansink and Misuru Shimizu, "Sports at Work."

have shown that former athletes typically earn more money than non-athletes. They also disproportionately had careers in upper management. So, you actually have the upper hand!

In fact, it may actually shock you once you join the workforce that many people lack the strengths that athletes develop to be successful. From the ability to go above and beyond for the good of the team to mental strength and multi-tasking, you'll soon realize, if you haven't already, that the strengths you've gained from sports can make you a better coworker, leader, and businessperson.

If you aren't feeling completely fulfilled by your new focus, I recommend getting involved with your athletic community. There are many coaching opportunities, perhaps at your alma mater, or for youth programs. You can also continue to participate in your sport recreationally. It wasn't until my husband started coaching his old high school basketball team that I realized how much I missed being part of the athletic atmosphere, and developing connections with other athletes. When I started personal training and helping athletes with nutrition, it made me feel like I was again connected to that world, helping athletes be the best and healthiest they can be—and that's the most fulfilling feeling I've ever had.

Getting What You Want: Meditation and Setting Intentions

Professional athletes, politicians, speakers, and performers commonly use intention setting and meditation exercises to build mental strength that aids in their success. If you cannot visualize what you want to happen, then you aren't really going anywhere. If you don't set goals—how do you know where you are headed?

> **TRANSITION PLAN**
> *Week Ten - Meditation & Setting Intentions*
> Practice this visualization technique to set your intentions and attract what you desire, whether it's for your day or future goals.

Take 10 to 15 minutes of your day for this visualization exercise each morning:

1. Take 10 to 15 minutes of your time to find a quiet place to sit and contemplate, preferably sitting or lying face up on a comfortable surface.
2. Close your eyes, and begin to notice your breath.
Also notice how your body feels. Start contemplating how your feet feel for several breaths, and then your ankles for several more breaths, your knees, and so on. Work your way up the body, all the way to your forehead.
3. Contemplate how it feels to be where you are for several breaths.
4. Get clear on what you want. You can focus on what you want to happen today, in the next week, month, or far into the future. Do you have a big interview coming up? Picture the interview going extremely well. Replay this in your head several times.
5. Next, imagine the physical senses of your vision. For example, what does it feel like to shake your future boss's hand or sit at your new desk? Think about how you want your life to look in five years. Picture what your current career is, where you are living, what your family looks like, how it makes you feel—everything from sights, smells,

THE ATHLETE AFTER

touch, and taste. Replay these visions several times.
6. Lastly, add in your emotions. Feel your elation as you get a promotion, or pride as you finish a big project. Replay these visions and feelings several times.
7. Come back to your body for several breaths and notice how you feel in this moment. Do not move right away. Slowly open your eyes, and sit until you feel ready to move.

All of us are living the Law of Attraction, every second of every day. The Law of Attraction can be understood as "like attracts like." Albert Einstein said, "Everything is energy, and that is all there is to it. Match the frequency of the reality you want, and you cannot help but get that reality. It can be no other way. This is not philosophy, this is physics."

It's also been discovered that energy vibrates, and due to the high intensity of its vibratory output, it creates, emits, and projects a measurable frequency. This means everyone and everything is made up of the same stuff, and what we are made of constantly emits frequency. The energy and frequency we emit, whether positive or negative, determines what we attract and experience. For example, if we spend our time wallowing in regrets of the past, or fearful of the future, you'll likely see more negativity appearing in your life. However, if you choose to see the positive in each experience, you'll notice more positivity surrounding you. We can choose how we use it, either consciously or unconsciously.

Those who understand this concept can utilize the energy and frequency they project in a conscious and intentional way to create desired experiences. Your thoughts, feelings, and emotions project a frequency as well. These frequencies are attracting frequencies that harmonize and attract whatever you are thinking and feeling. Consider your exercises on positive affirmations and self love—these thoughts will not only change your overall perception of happiness, but will also bring these thoughts and intentions into reality.

The quality of the thought is relevant. There is both low frequency and high frequency energy. The more intense the feeling or thought and emotions, the stronger the attraction. Perhaps reflect on your own life. Do you notice any patterns? They may appear in your friendships, relationships, finances, etc. These patterns can be tracked back to the type of energy we put out into the world and attract to us.

To attain what you want, start setting intentions. For example, if you noticed a negative pattern in your relationships, start thinking and imagining what it would feel like to have what you want instead. I have to admit this is how I found my husband and my career. After a pattern of failed relationships that seemed all-too-similar, I decided I wouldn't date someone who didn't fit exactly what I wanted in a partner. Not too long after I set that intention, Matt walked into my life. It was almost scary how much he met every single point on my list, and more.

When it came to my career, I realized after working behind a desk for the majority of my days that I needed something different to feel completely fulfilled. At the time I didn't know what that was, but I had a strong feeling that I had a purpose, and that I needed to feel like I was making a direct impact on someone's life. Then, I started seeing emails pop into my mailbox asking those very questions: Do you feel pulled to express your gifts and talents in ways that will make a difference, but have no idea how to realize your deeper potentials? Do you feel called to begin a new project or career that's about service and contribution, but don't know exactly what it might look like or how to support yourself in the meantime? Are you feeling uneasy and unfulfilled, and can't quite figure out why? It was a program to unlock feminine power to find true purpose.[31] I read it, and even tried to ignore it. But the emails kept coming, and I knew that I needed to follow the breadcrumbs. In that program I figured out that working with athletes to help them be healthy is what I'm here to do. I continue to set intentions and take the opportunities presented to me, and the rest is history. Working with other athletes again makes me feel like I'm living my purpose.

The Change in Relationships

Being identified as an athlete by others gives you a ticket into the inner-circle of sports. Within that circle are even more exclusive communities, depending on your sport. Because I was mainly a swimmer and basketball player in high school, I not only felt like I was part of my team, but that I could relate to other swimmers or basketball players I met. Beyond that, I felt even more kindred to those who swam long distance, and those who played in the post position on the court. We shared an understanding of long hours of training, sacrifice, injuries, winning, losing, etc., that comes with these sports and positions. You earn the right to be a runner, football player, gymnast—whatever it is. At the time, you may not even realize that these circles really exist. Or, you may understand that being a part of a team makes you feel like you are a part of something bigger than yourself.

---

[31] "The Three Keys to Feminine Power."

Regardless of how you feel when you are in the midst of it all, the strange reality is that after you conclude a certain sport, or leave a team, you may find yourself outside the circle and without the support system that was in place. The game continues without you there.

This can be devastating if you don't have other social circles, if the relationship with your family members was centered around your athletics, or if your coach was a main structure of support.

The surest way to avoid this is to try to develop relationships outside the circle of athletics and your team. I also encourage talking to other teammates who are making the transition at the same time, and helping to support each other in new ventures. Having an outlet for these struggles is important, and counseling can also be helpful. This is really where having a health coach can be beneficial. Having someone provide additional support in this transition can be critical to sorting through these changes.

Additional Support

The reality is that it can take longer than 10 weeks to gracefully make the transition from a full or part-time athlete to retirement, and/or a whole new career. The benefit in hiring a health coach to help is that they can be a pillar of support during this time, and can help you navigate these changes based on your individual needs.

A health coach is by definition a supportive mentor and

wellness authority who works with clients to help them feel their best through food and lifestyle changes, tailoring individualized wellness programs to meet their clients' needs.[32] One person may need more time spent specifically on diet, while another person may be trying to recover from the devastation of a career-ending injury. A coach can meet you where you are and provide the tools for a smooth transition.

> **TRANSITION PLAN**
> *Reflection*
> Take some time to reflect over the last 10 weeks. What have you learned about yourself? How has this program helped you? What additional support do you need?

You've had coaches guide you your whole life in how to improve and be successful at your sport. Why treat the rest of your life any differently?

These are some of the benefits of working one-on-one with a health coach:

- **Receive support and accountability in achieving your goals:** Working one-on-one, you receive guidance and support in taking the next steps for your own individual success.
- **Focus on your overall wellness:** From nutritional guidance and exercise programming to support and motivation, health coaches take a holistic approach to health and understand the science behind true behavior modification. We focus not just on the food that goes in your mouth, but also on everything else that nourishes you.

---

[32] "Nutrition and Health Coaching: The Health Coach."

This includes physical activity, career, relationships, and spirituality (whatever that means for you).
- **Overcome barriers:** There are a number of environmental and lifestyle factors that often serve as barriers to people trying to improve their overall health. Although obstacles are inevitable, with the right systems in place a health coach will arm you with the skills you need to cope with current and future difficulties.
- **Become self-reliant:** The ultimate goal of a health coach is to help you to become self-reliant—to listen to your body and understand what it needs.
- **Make it a lifestyle:** A health coach will empower you to take ownership of your experience and create positive, lasting lifestyle changes.

Group coaching can also be beneficial, especially to support teams in what they should be eating for their sport, or for a group of athletes who are transitioning out of their sport(s) together.

If you are interested in one-on-one, group, or team coaching, or to gain more information and tips, visit athleteafterword.com, join the community at facebook.com/athleteafter, and follow me on Twitter @athleteafter and Instagram @healthcoachk8e.

Univera: Essential Products for the Recovering Athlete

As a Certified Health Coaching and Personal Trainer, most clients come to me with the following issues:

- Joint discomfort, reduced mobility, and inflammation
- Digestive issues
- Lack of energy (over-caffeinated and stressed)

In addition, the recovering post-sport athlete typically suffers from chronic pain after years of training and stress. I struggled most with back pain. I was trying everything from chiropractic care, massage, and acupuncture. I continually searched for natural relief and started investigating natural products that could aid in the issues my clients and I experienced daily.

Thanks to the advice of fellow health coaches and trainers, I was introduced to the science of Univera. I found that Univera offered patented, plant-based formulas that quickly enhance cellular repair while decreasing cellular damage. I began recommending these products to clients with tremendous success. They were motivated to continue working out rather than feeling worn out. They soon reported improved joint-comfort and flexibility, increase mental clarity and focus, handled stress better, had improved digestive health, and more.

Whether current athletes are looking for faster recovery, post-sport athletes are looking to manage discomfort, or a client is simply looking to increase their metabolic health and reduce the affects of aging, Univera products provide many benefits in helping my clients reach their health and fitness goals.

For more information, visit www.univera.com/katiehargrave.

Becoming a Health Coach

This book was inspired by my experience at the Institute for Integrative Nutrition® (IIN), where I received my training in holistic wellness and health coaching.

IIN offers a truly comprehensive Health Coach Training Program that invites students to deeply explore the things that are most nourishing to them. From the physical aspects of nutrition and eating wholesome foods that work best for each individual person, to the concept of Primary Food—the idea that everything in life including our spirituality, career, relationships, and fitness contribute to our inner and outer health—IIN helped me reach optimal health and balance. This inner journey unleashed the passion that compelled me to share what I've learned and inspire others.

Beyond personal health, IIN offers training in health coaching, as well as business and marketing training. Students who choose to pursue this field professionally complete the program equipped with the communication skills and branding knowledge they need to create a fulfilling career by encouraging and supporting others to reach their own health goals.

From renowned wellness experts as visiting teachers to the convenience of their online learning platform, this school has changed my life and I believe it will do the same for you. I invite you to learn more about the Institute for Integrative Nutrition and explore how the Health Coach Training Program can help you transform your life. Learn more about my personal experience at athleteafterword.com, or call (844) 315-8546 to learn more.

References

Alfermann, Dorothee. "Causes and consequences of sport career termination." In Career Transition In Sport: International Perspectives, edited by David Lavallee and Paul Wylleman (2001): 45-58. doi: 10.1016/S1469-0292(02)00049-3

———. American Heart Association. "American Heart Association Recommendations for Physical Activity in Adults." Accessed February, 2014. http://www.heart.org/HEARTORG/Healthy Living/PhysicalActivity/FitnessBasics/American-Heart-Association-Recommendations-for-Physical-Activity-in-Adults

———. American Heart Association. "Know Your Fats." Accessed April 21, 2014. http://www.heart.org/HEARTORG/Conditions/Cholesterol/PreventionTreatmentofHighCholesterol/Know-Your-Fats

Blinde, Elaine, and Greendorfer, Susan. "A reconceptualization of the process of leaving the role of competitive athlete." In International Review for the Sociology of Sport (1985): 87-94. doi: 10.1177/101269028502000108

Brewer, Britton, VanRaalte, Judy, and Linder, Darwyn. "Athletic Identity: Hercules' muscles or Achilles heel?" International Journal of Sport Psychology (1993): 24, 237-254. https://www.researchgate.net/publication/232453451_Athletic_identity_Hercules'_muscles_or_Achilles_heel

Brewer, Britton, VanRaalte, Judy, and Linder, Darwyn. "Athletic Identity: Hercules' muscles or Achilles heel?" International Journal of Sport Psychology (1993): 24, 237-254. https://www.researchgate.net/publication/232453451_Athletic_identity_Hercules'_muscles_or_Achilles_heel

Bumgardner, Wendy. Verywell Fit. "Anaerobic vs. Aerobic Metabolism: Producing and Burning Energy for Exercise." Updated October 30, 2018. https://www.verywellfit.com/anaerobic-metabolism-3432629

Campbell, Bill, Krieder, Richard, Ziegenfuss, Tim, La Bounty, Paul, Roberts, Mike, Darren Burke, Landis, Jamie, Lopez, Hector and Antonio, Jose. "International Society of Sports Nutrition position stand: protein and exercise." In Journal of International Society of Sports Medicine (2007): doi 10.1186/1550-2783-4-8

———. Centers for Disease Control and Prevention. "AdultObesity Facts." Accessed August 6, 2016. https://www.cdc.gov/obesity/data/adult.html

Christensen, Jen. "FDA orders food manufacturers to stop using trans fat within three years." CNN.com, June 16, 2015: http://www.cnn.com/2015/06/16/health/fda-trans-fat/

Coakley, Stephany. "A phenomenological exploration of the sport-career transition experiences that affect subjective well-being of former National Football League players." Lecture at the University of North Carolina-Greensboro, 2006.

Couzens, Alan. "What type of athlete are you? Part Two: Your brain." Alancouzens.com, October 2, 2014: http://www.alancouzens.com blog/athlete_type_2.html

———. Dr. Fuhrman.com, Inc. "Nutrient Density." Accessed August 6, 2016. https://www.drfuhrman.com/learn/library/articles/55/nutrient-density

———. Feminine Power. "Feminine Power: The Essential Course for the Awakening Woman." http://femininepower.com/digital-course/ Accessed September 26, 2016.

———. The Impartial Guide to Endurance Training. "Fat Intake for Endurance Athletes." Accessed December 5, 2018. https://training4endurance.co.uk/nutrition/fat-intake-for-endurance-athletes

———. Harvard Medical School Department of Neurobiology. "Sugar and the Brain." Accessed August 6, 2016. http://neuro.hms.harvard.edu/harvard-mahoney-neuroscience-institute/brain-newsletter/and-brain-series/sugar-and-brain

Hoffman JR, Ratamess NA, Kang J, Falvo MJ, Faigenbaum AD. "Effect of protein intake on strength, body composition and endocrine changes in strength/power athletes." International Society of Sports Nutrition. 2006 Dec 13;3:12-8.

———. Institute for Integrative Nutrition. "Nutrition and Health Coaching: The Health Coach." Accessed August 30, 2016. http://www.integrativenutrition.com/health-coaching

Kleiber, Douglas, and Brock, Stephen. "The effect of career-ending injuries on the subsequent well-being of elite college athletes." In Sociology of Sport Journal (1992): 70-75. doi: 10.1123/ssj.9.1.70

Kniffin, Kevin, Wansink, Brian, and Shimizu, Misuru. "Sports at Work: Anticipated and Persistent Correlates of Participation in High School Athletics." In Journal of Leadership & Organizational Studies (May 2015): 217-230. doi:10.1177/1548051814538099

La Forge, Ralph. "Mind-Body Exercise," In American Council on Exercise Personal Trainer Manual, Fifth Edition (United States of America: American Council on Exercise United State of America, 2014): 480-482.

Lally, Patricia. "Identity and athletic retirement: A prospective study." In Psychology of Sport and Exercise (2007): 8, 85-99. doi: 10.1016/j.psychsport.2006.03.003

Lemon PW, Tarnopolsky MA, MacDougall JD, Atkinson SA. "Protein requirements and muscle mass/strength changes during intensive training in novice bodybuilders." Applied Physiology, 1992 Aug;73(2):767-75.

Lotysz, Greg, and Short, Sandra. "'What ever happened to . .': The effects of career termination from the national football league." In Athletic Insight: The Online Journal of Sport Psychology, 6(3). http://www.athleticinsight.com/Vol6Iss3/WhatEverHappened

———. Mayo Clinic. "Water: How much should you drink every day?" Accessed September 5, 2014. http://www.mayoclinic.org/healthy-lifestyle/nutrition-and-healthy-eating/in-depth/water/art

Ogilvie, Taylor, and Lavallee, David. "Career transition among athletes: Is there life after sports?" In Applied Sport Psychology: Personal Growth to Peak Performance, edited by Williams, J.M. (1998): 429-444.

Olson, Richard, Casavale, Kellie, Rihane, Colette, Essery Stoody, Eve, Britten, Patricia, Reedy, Jill, Rahavi, Elizabeth, et al. Dietary Guidelines for Americans 2015-2020, Eighth Edition, edited by Anne Brown Rodgers.

———. Online Casino. "The Odds of Success." Accessed August 6, 2016. https://www.onlinecasino.ca/odds-of-success

Payne, Marissa. "So you want to be a pro athlete? You might not get paid well." The Washington Post, October 29, 2014. https://www.washingtonpost.com/news/early-lead/wp/2014/10/29/so-you-want-to-be-a-pro-athlete-you-might-not-get-paid-well/

Pearson, Richard, and Petitpas, Albert. "Transitions of athletes: Developmental and preventive perspectives." In Journal of Counseling & Development (1990): 7-19. doi: 10.1002/j.1556-6676.1990.tb01445.x

Scheett, Stoppani, and McGuigan, Michael. "NSCA Sports Nutrition Education Program." NSCA National Strength and Conditioning Association. Accessed December 5, 2018. https://macalester_ftp.sidearmsports.com/custompages/Deno_Videos/nutrition/nutrition_for_strength_and_power_athletes.pdf

Shilhavy, Brian. "Time Magazine: We Were Wrong About Saturated Fats. But Don't Expect More Mainstream Media to Follow this Repentance on Saturated Fats." Health Impact News, 2014. https://healthimpactnews.com/2014/time-magazine-we-were-wrong-about-saturated-fats/

Sisson, Mark. "The Primal Blueprint: An Evolution-Based High-Performance Eating Strategy." Lecture at Institute for Integrative Nutrition, New York, New York.

Stephan, Yannick, Bilard, Jean, Ninot, Gregory and Delignieres, Didier. "Repercussions of transition out of elite sport on subjective well-being: a one year study." In Journal of Applied Sport Psychology (2003): 354-371. doi: 10.1080/714044202

Sweeney, Michael, and Green, Cynthia. Complete Guide to Brain Health: How to Stay Sharp, Improve Memory, and Boost Creativity. Washington D.C.: National Geographic Society, 2013.

Tarnopolsky, M. A., Atkinson, S. A., MacDougall, J. D., Chesley, A., Phillips, S., & Schwarcz, H. P. "Evaluation of protein requirements for trained strength athletes." Journal of Applied Physiology, (1992) 73(5), 1986-1995.

——— . University of Maryland Medical Center. "Omega-3 Fatty Acids." Accessed August 5, 2015. http://umm.edu/health/medical/altmed/supplement/omega3-fatty-acids

Westcott, Wayne. "Resistance Training." In American Council on Exercise Personal Trainer Manual, Fifth Edition (United States of America: American Council on Exercise, 2014): 329.

Wylleman, Paul, Alfermann, Dorothee, and Lavallee, David. "Career transitions in sport: European perspectives." In Psychology of Sport and Exercise (2004): 5, 7-20. doi: 10.1016/S1469-0292(02)00049-3

Zeratsky, Katherine. Mayo Clinic Healthy Lifestyle: Nutrition and Healthy Eating. "To track how much fat I eat each day, should I focus on grams, calories or percentages?" Accessed December 5, 2018. https://mayoclinic.org/healthy-lifestyle/nutrition-and-healthy-eating/expert-answers/fat-grams/faq-20058496

TRANSITION PLAN

POST-SPORT ATHLETE TRANSITION PLAN

This workbook is meant to serve as an individualized transition plan, to be used while reading this book. I advise filling out one section per week as recommended to give yourself enough time to notice change and reflect. It can take longer than 10 weeks to make lasting changes, but this book and plan are a good start!

Week One - Food Tracking

Find a food-tracking app (FitBit, MyFitnessPal, and LoseIt are the most popular). Eat and drink as you usually would and start tracking your intake. It's important to establish your baseline so you can identify where to make adjustments. In your plan, note how you feel throughout the day. How's your energy? Do you feel strong, weak, tired, or hungry? Do you have a headache, nausea, or constipation? Be detailed. You'll be surprised by what patterns might stick out to you. At the end of the week, average out how many calories you are injesting, as well as how many grams of protein and carbohydrates.

Day 1:
_____
_____

Day 2:
_____
_____

Day 3:
_____
_____

Day 4:
_____
_____

Day 5:
_____
_____

Day 6:
_____
_____

Day 7:
_____
_____

Protein Average_____
Carbohydrate Average_____
Fat Average_____
Calorie Average_____

Week Two - Water

If you are currently not big on water intake, start by aiming for 64 ounces per day. If you are already getting this much, target drinking half your body weight in ounces. Each day,

TRANSITION PLAN

write down the number of ounces consumed and how you felt throughout the day.

Body weight / 2 = _____ ounces of water per day.

Other suggestions:

Try drinking a glass of water first thing in the morning. When you wake up from sleep, your body is naturally dehydrated. This is why drinking coffee first further dehydrates you. Your body is also repairing itself while you sleep, so drinking water immediately upon waking helps flush toxins out. It also fires up your metabolism, fuels your brain, and relieves constipation.

When you're hungry for a snack, try drinking a glass of water first. Dehydration often causes a feeling of hunger.

Day 1: _____ ounces

_____

_____

Day 2: _____ ounces

_____

_____

Day 3: _____ ounces

_____

_____

Day 4: _____ ounces

_____

_____

THE ATHLETE AFTER

Day 5: _____ ounces

_____

_____

Day 6: _____ ounces

_____

_____

Day 7: _____ ounces

_____

_____

~~~~~~~~~~~~~~~~~~~~~~~~

Week Three - Macronutrients

Now that you know what's in your every-day food, set your macro and calorie goals below and in your food tracker. Consider what you need to change to stay within those zones this week. As you go, continue to track how you feel each day. Do you recognize any changes? Average out your macro nutrients and calories at the end of the week, and see how close you were to meeting your goals.

Protein Goal

Body Weight _____ x _____ g = _____ g protein per day
Losing fat or gaining muscle (0.6-0.9g), maintaining weight (0.5g)

Total protein _____ g / by 5 = approx. _____ g at each meal
Meals: breakfast, lunch, pre workout, post workout, dinner

TRANSITION PLAN

Carbohydrate Goal _____ g per day (not counting fiber)
Weight loss 50-100g per day, weight maintenance 100-150g per day

Fat and Calorie Goal

Fat goal range _____ % of calories per day
Weight loss 20-25%, strength/power training 25-30%,
endurance training 30-35%

Protein _____ g (minimum goal from above) x 4 calories per gram = _____ calories per day in protein minimum

Carbohydrate _____ g (minimum goal from above) x 4 calories per gram = _____ calories per day in carbohydrates minimum

Protein calories _____ + carbohydrate calories _____ = _____ calories for both protein and carbohydrates per day

Combined total of protein and carbohydrate calories _____ divided by inverse of minimum percentage of fat goal (for example, divide by .75 if your goal is 25% of your calories from fat per day minimum) = _____ total minimum calories per day

Total minimum calories per day _____ minus combined protein and carbohydrate calories per day = _____ minimum calories from fat per day

Total minimum calories from fat per day _____ divided by 9 calories of fat per gram = _____ g of fat per day minimum

THE ATHLETE AFTER

Repeat process with maximum numbers to get your range for fat and calories.

Protein _____ g (maximum goal from above) x 4 calories per gram = _____ calories per day in protein maximum

Carbohydrate _____ g (maximum goal from above) x 4 calories per gram = _____ calories per day in carbohydrates maximum

Protein calories _____ + carbohydrate calories _____ = _____ calories for both protein and carbohydrates per day

Combined total of protein and carbohydrate calories _____ divided by inverse of maximum percentage of fat goal (for example, divide by .75 if your goal is 25% of your calories from fat per day maximum) = _____ total maximum calories per day

Total maximum calories per day _____ minus combined protein and carbohydrate calories per day = _____ maximum calories from fat per day

Total maximum calories from fat per day _____ divided by 9 calories of fat per gram = _____ g of fat per day maximum

Range of fat per day in grams _____ g
Range in calories per day based on above macronutrient goals
_____

TRANSITION PLAN

Day 1:
_____
_____

Day 2:
_____
_____

Day 3:
_____
_____

Day 4:
_____
_____

Day 5:
_____
_____

Day 6:
_____
_____

Day 7:
_____
_____

Protein Average_____
Carbohydrate Average_____
Fat Average_____
Calorie Average_____

Week Four - Food Adjustment

Evaluate and tweak your meals based on how you felt last week. Did you feel really full or tired at certain times of the day? Look back at what you ate the previous meal and consider what could have made you feel that way. Experiment with different types of protein. Do you need more energy to sustain your workout? Add a few more carbohydrates to your pre-workout snack. Are you feeling low on energy and unfocused around 3:00-4:00 pm? Look at what you had for lunch, and adjust to eat fewer carbohydrates and, perhaps, add more fat and protein. Choosing your fuel based on how your body feels is more important than hitting your exact macro goals—these are just a guideline.

Day 1:

Day 2:

Day 3:

Day 4:

Day 5:

TRANSITION PLAN

Day 6:
_____
_____

Day 7:
_____
_____

Protein Average_____
Carbohydrate Average_____
Fat Average_____
Calorie Average_____

What have you taken away from this last month of tracking and adjusting your food and water intake? Take some time to reflect in the following prompts.

Did you notice changes in your energy?
_____
_____
_____

Did you notice changes in your mood?
_____
_____
_____

Did you notice changes in your overall digestion?
_____
_____
_____

Did you notice changes in your focus and mental clarity?
_____
_____
_____

Did you notice changes in your sleep?
_____
_____
_____

What other changes did you notice?
_____
_____
_____

Post what you noticed at facebook.com/athleteafter.

~~~~~~~~~~~~~~~~~~~~~~~~~~~

Week Five - Micronutrient Focus

You should now feel more comfortable eating within your macronutrient ranges. Now, try incorporating more micronutrients from Dr. Fuhrman's list of G-BOMBS. Where can you fit in more greens, beans, onions, mushrooms, berries, and seeds? Try to include them in your daily diet. Circle what you were able to incorporate and how you did it, and if you noticed any change in how you feel.

Day 1:   Greens   Beans   Onions   Mushrooms   Berries   Seeds
_____
_____

TRANSITION PLAN

Day 2:   Greens   Beans   Onions   Mushrooms   Berries   Seeds

_____

Day 3:   Greens   Beans   Onions   Mushrooms   Berries   Seeds

_____

Day 4:   Greens   Beans   Onions   Mushrooms   Berries   Seeds

_____

Day 5:   Greens   Beans   Onions   Mushrooms   Berries   Seeds

_____

Day 6:   Greens   Beans   Onions   Mushrooms   Berries   Seeds

_____

Day 7:   Greens   Beans   Onions   Mushrooms   Berries   Seeds

_____

Protein Average_____
Carbohydrate Average_____
Fat Average_____
Calorie Average_____

THE ATHLETE AFTER

Week Six - Physical Activity

One of the key components to a consistent exercise routine is accountability. As athletes, we were once held accountable by coaches and teammates. Now, we have to rely on something else: a friend, trainer, or simply our own willpower. Regardless of how you stay accountable, tracking your progress will also help keep you on target.

As you plan out your exercise for the week, refer to the American Heart Association (AHA) recommendations for exercise on page 54. Incorporate different types of exercise, like walking, weight lifting, and/or hiking on the weekend.

Type of Exercise	Day 1	Day 2	Day 3	Day 4	Day 5	Day 6	Day 7

Total minutes of light activity this week:_____
Total minutes of moderate activity this week:_____
Total minutes of intense activity this week:_____
Total minutes of muscle strengthening activity this week:_____

Note how you feel after different types of activity. Just as everyone is an individual with the type of food that feels best, everyone is an individual with which activity feels best. Experiment to discover what works for you.

TRANSITION PLAN

What did you notice about the activities you tried this week?
_____
_____
_____

How did exercise impact your energy level and quality of sleep?
_____
_____
_____

How did exercise affect your eating habits, and the other way around?
_____
_____
_____

How do workouts in the morning compare to evening exercise?
_____
_____
_____

~~~~~~~~~~~~~~~~~~~~~~~~~~~~

Week Seven - Exercise Goals

Now that you've started scheduling your exercise and recognizing how it makes you feel, start thinking about goals that will keep you motivated. You've also read different types of activities may be best for you, depending on where you are on the scale of reactivity. Identify what you are, and start trying activities that fit within your classification. Then, start setting goals that will keep you motivated, whether it is to finish your first bicycle tour, run a mile every morning, or join a group training class.

Chart by Athletic Type Based on Dopamine and Seratonin Levels

Volume →

High Reactive/Low Response Does well with high frequency, high volume, low intensity modes of activity	Low Reactive/Low Response Does well with varied stimuli of mixed intensity.
	Low Reactive/High Response Does well with short bouts of focused and intense work.

Intensity →

My Reactivity/Response Type: _____

Goal: _____
_____

To be accomplished by: _____

Goal: _____
_____

To be accomplished by: _____

Goal: _____
_____

To be accomplished by: _____

TRANSITION PLAN

Now, tailor your weekly activities to reach these goals.

Type of Exercise	Day 1	Day 2	Day 3	Day 4	Day 5	Day 6	Day 7

Again, note how you felt this week after your activities.

What did you notice about the activities you tried this week?
___
___

How did exercise impact your energy level and quality of sleep?
___
___

How did exercise affect your eating habits, and the other way around?
___
___

How do workouts in the morning compare to evening exercise?
___
___

Post what you noticed at facebook.com/athleteafter.

Week Eight - Self Love

One of the most difficult parts of the post-athlete transition, especially for female athletes, is accepting the changes in our bodies. "Perfect" abs, legs, and arms are plastered all over the media demonstrating today's beauty ideals. These ideal standards are difficult to get away from, especially when we didn't have to work hard outside of training to maintain this type of body in the not-so-distant past.

The trick to loving and appreciating yourself is realizing that your body is a wonderful, amazing, beautiful encasement of your soul. We were given one body to have the ability to experience this amazing life. Treat yourself like the amazing being that you are!

List 10 reasons you are thankful for your body:

1._____
_____

2._____
_____

3._____
_____

4._____
_____

5._____
_____

TRANSITION PLAN

6._____

_____

7._____

_____

8._____

_____

9._____

10._____

_____

This week, every time you see yourself in a mirror, tell yourself you are beautiful.

Write a positive affirmation and post it in three different places you will see constantly (examples include the background of your phone, in your wallet, on your mirror, etc.).

Some tips for writing a great affirmation:
- An affirmation should always be stated as if the desired outcome is already happening or has happened (use the present or past tense).
- Use the most positive words you can think of.
- Keep it short and specific. It will be easier to remember.

Some examples:
- I am beautiful in my own skin.
- I am grateful for who I am.
- My imperfections are uniquely perfect in their own way.

THE ATHLETE AFTER

Affirmation:
_____
_____

I will post it:
1._____
2._____
3._____

At the end of every day this week, write one thing you love about yourself.

Day 1:
_____
_____

Day 2:
_____
_____

Day 3:
_____
_____

Day 4:
_____
_____

Day 5:
_____
_____

TRANSITION PLAN

Day 6:
_____
_____

Day 7:
_____
_____

~~~~~~~~~~~~~~~~~~~~~~~~~~~~~

Week Nine - Channeling Your Skillset

Your strengths that have made you a successful athlete can be channeled into a successful and fulfilling career.

Write down six non-physical qualities that make you good at your sport:

Examples: team-player, leader, competitive, strategic, etc.

1. _____
2. _____
3. _____
4. _____
5. _____
6. _____

Write down six physical qualities that make you good at your sport:

Examples: powerful, fast, intimidating, strong, etc.

THE ATHLETE AFTER

7. _____
8. _____
9. _____
10. _____
11. _____
12. _____

Results from Tony Robbins' DISC Survey:

First, take the survey at tonyrobbins.com/ue/. Read through your results and answer the following questions.

Do you feel the four components of behavior fit your personality style?

Decisive

_____
_____

Interactive

_____
_____

Stabilizing

_____
_____

Cautious

_____
_____

Reflect on your current career choice, non-physical and physical qualities, as well as your results from the DISC survey. Write

TRANSITION PLAN

down how your unique qualities can make you successful in your current job.

1. _____
2. _____
3. _____
4. _____
5. _____
6. _____
7. _____
8. _____
9. _____
10. _____

Again, reflecting on your individual need for motivation and ideal work climate, list six things you need/needed from teammates and/or coaches to feel successful.

1. _____
2. _____
3. _____
4. _____
5. _____

THE ATHLETE AFTER

6. _____

How do these apply to your current career?

1. _____

2. _____

3. _____

4. _____

5. _____

6. _____

Take a moment to review your answers to the questions above. Are you having a hard time relating your skillset to your current job? Are you able to get the feedback, support, acknowledgment, or whatever it is you need from your coworkers and/or boss? Depending on your answers, it may be time to consider what your overall career goals are, and how you can best reach them. You may find your current career is not the right fit for you. Or, you may realize you are in the right job, but aren't utilizing your behavioral styles to support your success.

TRANSITION PLAN

Week Ten - Meditation and Setting Intentions

Every day this week, set aside 10 to 15 minutes to do the following visualization exercise on page 75. Before you begin, write out what you desire to happen, whether it is in your immediate future or further down the road. This will help prevent you from getting into a meditative state without a point of focus. Some examples of focus points:

A.) Picture yourself in your dream job. What does it look like? Do you have an office? Are you working from home? How much money do you make? What makes you the happiest about your job?

B.) Decide you are going to have a great day. Imagine yourself feeling great, accomplishing everything you need to do, including your interactions, what your meals are like, etc.

Day 1:
_____
_____

Day 2:
_____
_____

Day 3:
_____
_____

Day 4:
_____
_____

Day 5:
_____
_____

Day 6:
_____
_____

Day 7:
_____
_____

~~~~~~~~~~~~~~~~~~~~~~~~~~~

Reflection

Now that you have finished the book and 10-week program to a balanced lifestyle post-sport, reflect on what you have discovered. How have your food choices changed? How do you feel in your body? What have you learned about yourself? Write some notes below.

After finishing the Food section of the program, I learned:
_____
_____
_____

After finishing the Body section of the program, I learned:
_____
_____
_____

TRANSITION PLAN

After finishing the Mind section of the program, I learned:
_____
_____
_____

The most significant overall change I've noticed in myself has been:
_____
_____

The most significant piece of information I learned was:
_____
_____

I still feel like I need to work on:
_____
_____

I will continue to work on this by:
_____
_____

Congratulations on completing the 10-week Transition Plan! My hope is that you have gained valuable takeaways that have improved your transition into a healthier overall lifestyle.

While the reality is that it can take longer than 10 weeks to gracefully make the transition from a full or part-time athlete to retirement and/or a whole new career, 10 weeks is an amazing start.

THE ATHLETE AFTER

If you are interested in one-on-one, group, or team coaching, or to gain more information and tips, visit athleteafterword.com, join the community at facebook.com/athleteafter, and follow me on Twitter @athleteafter and Instagram @healthcoachk8e.

TRANSITION PLAN

Notes

Manufactured by Amazon.ca
Bolton, ON